MW01711252

Rheumatoid Arthritis: The Alternate Route

by

Susanne Harris, Ph.D.

Rheumatoid Arthritis:

The Alternate Route

by

Susanne Harris

Cover design by Renny James

ISBN 1-932196-87-0

One Night Books
#6

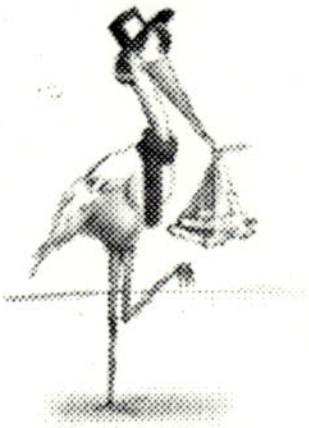

WordWright.biz, Inc.

WordWright Business Park

46561 State Highway 118

Alpine, TX 79830

Printed in the United States of America

Table of Contents

For my Mum, Judith

Thank you for teaching me to be a strong,
independent woman
and for showing me how to survive
in a world full of pain.
Without you,
I would never have found the inner strength
to fight my illness.
I will hold you in my heart always.
I love you, mum.

Acknowledgments

I'd like to thank all the people who have helped make this book possible, especially my mum who guided me through some of the most painful times of my life. Without her strength and determination to make me fight my illness, I'd have given up a long time ago.

My husband, Mark, whose constant support gives me the push I need to take life by the horns and shake it, and for not allowing me to fall into the destructive blackness of self-pity. Thank you for loving me.

I also wish to offer my thanks to my surgeon who gave me my life back after the years I spent in a wheelchair. Without his knowledge and dedication I'd still sit in that wheelchair, instead of walking and living a full and happy life.

My unending gratitude to my friend, Pamela Duff, whose invaluable advice and research helped me enormously in formulating this handbook. In fact, thank you to all who gave their time to contribute and advise in order to help others. They are numerous and too many to list, but they know who they are.

My publisher, Joan R. Neubauer, whose patience, guidance and input helped make this book what it is today. I could not have done it without you. Thank you for believing in me.

Finally, yet equally importantly, my children; their

patience and understanding that I cannot do things as quickly as I might, helps make my life easier; especially when the illness flares up and the pain grows unbearable.

Foreword

We use Rheumatoid Arthritis as a comprehensive term for a decidedly individualistic disease when it comes to cause and course of action. Conventional medicine follows a narrow course in the treatment of RA -- alleviate pain, reduce inflammation, and slow down joint damage. We accomplish this with the use of painkillers and steroids. When those fail, surgery becomes the final option. But this presents a problem. Nature uses pain to tell us something's wrong. After you numb the pain, you still have the problem. Only now it gets worse because the damage continues at an accelerated rate, since the warning sign, pain, has been removed. Furthermore, conventional medicine gives little thought to reversing the course of a disease or even preventing it from occurring. In fact, doctors generally consider such ideas impossible, if not absurd.

For thousands of years, alternative therapies made up the standard form of treatment, but for less than one century, we've been conditioned to believe that modern medicine provides superior care and we should heed only that. Tragically, the world witnesses the futility of such rigid beliefs. But all is not lost, as many in the medical community grow interested in a blended variety of treatments to manage health concerns rather than unrealistically hoping for a supposed universal cure. We just now see what one wise British physician once visualized:

"The work of the doctor will, in the future, be ever more that of an educator, and ever less that of a man who treats ailments." (Lord Horder, physician to five successive British monarchs from Edward VII to Elizabeth II)

As a registered nurse, I saw many cases of arthritis in its cruellest forms. I watched as conventional treatments did little more than mask the symptoms. However, these methods often created even more problems, especially with liver and kidney functions. For more than thirty-five years, the field of nutrition has fascinated me, ever since I saw it correct a condition our oldest son had at the time. That should not have come as such a surprise to me, but it did.

Over 2,400 years ago, Hippocrates, the father of modern medicine, said, "Let food be thy medicine and let thy medicine be food." When we continually inundate our body with foods it cannot process, and we consistently ignore the messages our body sends us, the body responds in the form of a disease or disorder. It becomes apparent that, if diet and lifestyle practices exacerbated a problem, elimination should diminish the problem. I tested this reasoning with family and friends, and in my patient teaching, those willing to try found good results.

Since we recognize RA as a complication of a chronic digestive disorder, I reasoned that diet should make up an essential part in its prevention or reversal. I observed that certain foods aggravate the conditions of some but not others. As I studied these diet phenomena, I identified food allergies, or sensitivities, as major factors in the development and speedy progression of many diseases. As I watched my father suffer with arthritis, I helped him only a little, by teaching him which foods and medicines aggravated his condition, and which ones eased the symptoms without harming the rest of his body.

Suzanne Harris helps to push the quest for a wider

variety of RA treatments by writing this timely book. Since RA affects people differently, she describes what has worked for her and what she has found in her research. Each individual must assume responsibility to find a treatment that helps him/her and then share that knowledge with others.

Suzanne researched carefully. Take her suggestions, investigate them for yourself, try them, analyze the advantages and disadvantages of all available treatments, seek alternative measures, determine if previous studies have been done on them, and ask others what works for them. Do all that you can do to heal yourself. No one else cares as much about your health as much as you do.

I wish you well in your search. You will find that it is truly an exciting and rewarding learning experience.

Pamela Duff, Registered Nurse.
Canada

Introduction

Can you imagine being seven years old, active, and suddenly struck down by terrible pain? I found myself in that situation. I went from a "normal," happy child to one who slept all the time and cried because of the pains in my legs. My mother took me to doctors, concerned at the way I rapidly lost interest in life. It took six years to get a clinical diagnosis (after several attempts with them trying to convince her I suffered growing pains) only to hear I had Chronic Juvenile Rheumatoid Arthritis and that I'd grow out of it. I am now thirty-five and still waiting to grow out of it. However, I've managed to control it.

After years of downing anti-inflammatory drugs, painkillers, aspirin and steroids and taking gold injections, all to no avail, I ended up at twenty-three wheelchair bound and told that I was too young to operate on. Therefore, I dealt with the problem directly and changed my own life by gradually coming off all my medication.

I must emphasize, however, *you should never attempt to do this yourself and certainly not without consulting your physician first as it could prove dangerous to stop any medication. Always do it under medical guidance as any decision to come off your drugs should be very carefully considered and done gradually to avoid the risk of withdrawal symptoms.* Eventually, at age thirty, I had my knee replaced, managed to get back on my feet and then gradually, and systematically, I changed my whole life.

This book will guide you through that journey as I share all the knowledge I gained along the way. I have also included plenty of information about nutrition, exercise, latest alternative therapies and advice from experts who will all help you to change your life and feel pain-free, and healthier, more often. There are recipes you can quickly prepare, none taking more than thirty minutes. They taste good and provide nutrition. Although the medical profession shuns many of these therapies by saying no proven research backs the claims made by the manufacturers of the products, many people swear by the health benefits they've found. I myself have tried many of the products in this book and can honestly say I now feel relatively pain-free and completely free of conventional drugs. I do not take steroids or NSAIDs anymore, and I feel much better for it.

Arthritis normally strikes in the thirties or forties and women who suffer from it outnumber men three-to-one, but as you can see, even young people can develop it. I did. No matter what your age, background or social standing we all risk developing this crippling disease, making it even more important that we eat properly, take regular vitamin supplements and stay active. It does not guarantee you will be arthritis-free, but it will help you stay healthier, making you less susceptible to a whole host of diseases, not just arthritis. Get ready to change your life.

Chapter 1

What is Arthritis?

Medical professionals use the term "arthritis" to describe the inflammation of joints. According to statistics recorded on the University of Virginia health system website, Rheumatoid Arthritis is the most crippling form of arthritis. It currently affects approximately 2.1 million Americans (500,000 British) and two to three times more women than men. The average onset for the disease is between the ages of twenty and forty-five years old. However, the disease now affects more people in their twenties and thirties than ever before. Arthritis Foundation studies reveal that it costs the U.S. economy 65 billion dollars per year in medical care directly and indirectly, such as lost wages and lost production costs. In the U.K. this disease costs 5.5 billion dollars. This pattern is mirrored the world over.

What is Rheumatoid Arthritis?

Rheumatoid Arthritis, or RA, is a type of inflammatory arthritis and an autoimmune disorder, caused when the body turns on itself. An overactive immune system can harm you as much as a weak one. This happens when the body's immune system improperly identifies the synovial membrane as foreign and begins attacking it. This antigen response results in inflammation and damaged cartilage and tissues in and around the joints.

The following sentence will not be clear to the lay person, but I don't know how to clarify it. Perhaps the writer will consider a different explanation. Candidates for a precipitating antigen include three groups of infectious microorganisms: bacteria, mycoplasmas, and viruses, especially the Epstein-Barr virus. With long-term or intensive exposure to the antigen, normal antibodies become autoantibodies, or antibodies that attack the host tissue. Because they are usually present in those with RA, we call these transformed antibodies rheumatoid factors (RFs), which aggregate, or group, into complexes and generate inflammation.

Causes of RA point to infections, genetic predispositions and endocrine factors. Experts believe that genetic susceptibility develops when an abnormal, or altered IgG antibodies, are exposed to an antigen and then passed on. Whichever offending organism causes the damage, those genetically susceptible end up with the joint lining becoming inflamed, especially the part that meets the cartilage. Over time, chronic inflammation makes the joint lining thick and overgrown, which then begins to invade the cartilage, other joint-supporting tissues, and even the bone, weakening the entire structure. Eventually, the weakened joint becomes more painful and less able to perform. Pressure may even dislocate and deform it.

RA particularly frustrates us because of spontaneous remissions and unpredictable exacerbations. It hits suddenly, usually appearing in the same joint on both sides of the body. In its mildest form, RA is characterized by joint discomfort, but in the more severe cases, it causes painfully deformed joints and harms body organ systems. Of RA patients, about 10 percent will have a single episode followed by a spontaneous long-term remission. The other

90 percent will suffer from chronic joint inflammation with occasional flare-ups, but the disease becomes progressively worse over time.

Since Rheumatoid Arthritis is a chronic systemic disease affecting the body's connective tissues, we also classify it as a collagen disease. The first joint tissue it affects is the synovial membrane. This soon spreads to the articular cartilage, joint capsule, and surrounding ligaments and tendons, causing pain, deformity, and loss of function. It most commonly affects joints in the fingers, feet, wrists, elbows, ankles, and knees, but the shoulders, hips, and cervical spine may become involved. Affected joints stiffen after an activity or rest, especially first thing in the morning.

If the disease actively progresses, look for deformities. The fingers may become fixed in a characteristic "swan's neck" or "boutonniere" deformity from marked oedema and congestion in the joints. The hands appear foreshortened, the wrists boggy. Carpal tunnel syndrome may develop from synovial pressure on the median nerve, causing tingling in the fingers. The most common finding, outside the joints, is the gradual appearance of rheumatoid nodules (subcutaneous, round or oval nontender masses), usually on such pressure areas as the elbows.

Besides joint inflammation, RA can cause fever, malaise, rash, lymph node or spleen enlargement, and Raynaud's phenomenon, a lack of circulation to the fingers and toes. Along with the swollen, tender, and inflamed joints, the sufferer may lose weight and generally feel sick, sore, stiff, and achy. The eyes and mouth dry out if RA involves the tear and salivary glands. Patients often appear undernourished and chronically ill. Most suffer anaemia because of the effect of the disease on blood-forming organs.

Stages of RA

Joint change generally occurs in four general stages, but along with these appear the atrophy of muscles, bones, and skin adjacent to the affected joint.

- **Stage One:** Synovitis develops from congestion and oedema of the synovial membrane and joint capsule.
- **Stage Two:** Formation of pannus occurs, covering the cartilage and eventually destroying the joint capsule and bone.
- **Stage Three:** Fibrous ankylosis, a fibrous invasion of pannus and scar tissue that fills the joint space, occurs. Bone atrophy and mal-alignment cause visible deformities and disrupt the articulation of opposing bones. This, in turn, causes muscle atrophy and imbalance that may include partial dislocations (subluxations).
- **Stage Four:** Fibrous tissue begins to calcify, resulting in bony ankylosis (total immobility).

Path physiology of RA

Rheumatoid Factors (RFs) usually consist of two classes of immunoglobulin antibodies -- antibodies for IgM and IgG (occasionally IgA). They mainly target portions of the immunoglobulin molecule. RFs bind with their target self-antigens in the blood and synovial membrane, forming immune complexes (antigen-antibody). Synovial inflammation (synovitis) occurs when the immune complexes in blood and synovial tissue trigger the inflammatory response by activating the plasma protein complement. This stimulation activates kinin and prostaglandin release that increases the permeability of blood vessels in the synovial membranes. This attracts several types of leukocytes and lymphocytes to the synovial membrane out of the circulation.

The phagocytes of inflammation (neutrophils and macrophages) ingest the immune complexes, which releases powerful enzymes that degrade synovial tissue and articular cartilage. The immune system's B and T lymphocytes are also activated. The B lymphocytes produce more RFs, and the T lymphocytes produce enzymes that increase the inflammatory response. A microorganism, which may originally be responsible, can be killed off and removed from the body. However, in an autoimmune response, the newly targeted self-antigens (immunoglobulin perpetuate indefinitely the formation of immune complexes.

Inflammatory and immune processes damage the synovial membrane in several ways. Inflammation causes haemorrhage, coagulation, and fibrin deposits on the synovial membrane, in the intracellular matrix, and in the synovial fluid. Over denuded areas of the synovial membrane, fibrin develops into granulation tissue called pannus, the earliest tissue produced in the healing process. Researchers disagree about whether pannus is a cause or an effect of articular cartilage involvement in RA. Some believe that, as the disease progresses, pannus extends from the synovial membrane into adjacent articular cartilage and destroys the cartilage. Others think that pannus forms on articular cartilage after inflammation destroys the cartilage. In any case, pannus formation does not lead to synovial or articular regeneration, but rather to formation of scar tissue that immobilizes the joint.

Along with the swelling caused by leukocyte infiltration, the synovial membrane undergoes hyperplasic thickening as its cells abnormally proliferate and enlarge. As synovial inflammation progresses to involve its blood vessels, small venules (a tiny vessel that collects blood from the capillaries and joins to form veins) become occluded by hypertrophied endothelial cells, fibrin, platelets, and inflammatory cells. These vascular derangements decrease blood flow to the synovial tissue and compromised circulation. This, coupled with increased metabolic needs due to hypertrophy and hyperplasia, causes hypoxia (oxygen depletion) and metabolic acidosis. Acidosis stimulates the release of hydrolytic enzymes from synovial cells into the surrounding tissue, initiating erosion of the articular cartilage, and inflammation spreads into the supporting ligaments and tendons.

Diagnosing RA

- **X-rays:** In the early stages, X-rays will show bone demineralization and soft-tissue swelling. Later, they show loss of cartilage and the narrowing of joint spaces. Finally, they will show cartilage and bone destruction, erosion, subluxations, and deformities.
- **RF test:** The Rheumatoid Factor test will come back positive in about 80% of the patients, as indicated by a titre of 1:160 or higher.
- **Synovial fluid analysis:** This test will show increased volume and turbidity but a decrease in viscosity and complement (C3 and C4) levels. WBCs (white blood cells) will often be more than 10,000/mm.
- **Serum protein electrophoresis:** This test may show elevated serum globulins.
- **Erythrocyte sedimentation rate:** It is elevated in 85-90 percent of patients. It may be useful in monitoring response to therapy, since an elevation frequently parallels disease activity.
- **CBC:** A complete blood count will usually indicate moderate anaemia and slight leukocytosis in the RA patient.

Complications of RA

One major complication is vasculitis, or inflammation of a vessel, which can lead to skin lesions or cysts, leg ulcers, and multiple systemic complications. The formation of cysts in the articular cartilage or subchondral bone occasionally communicates with the skin surface, usually the sole of the foot, and can drain through passages called fistulas. Thromboses of these vessels may lead to heart attacks, strokes, kidney damage, and vascular insufficiency in the hands and fingers (Raynaud's phenomenon), which may produce numbness or tingling in the feet or weakness and loss of sensation in the fingers. We see vascular changes primarily in individuals receiving steroid therapy. Thus, we believe the therapy plays a role in initiating these lesions.

Rheumatoid nodules may also invade the skin, cardiac valves, pericardium, pleura, lung parenchyma, and spleen. These nodules appear identical to those encountered in some individuals with rheumatic fever and are characterized by central tissue necrosis surrounded by proliferating connective tissue. Also, we see large numbers of lymphocytes and occasional plasma cells. The skin nodules appear in about 20 percent of those affected with RA, mostly involving the arms and elbows. Less commonly they appear on the scalp, back, hands, feet, buttocks, and knees.

Acute glaucoma may result with nodules forming on the sclera. Pulmonary involvement may result in diffuse pleuritis or multiple intraparenchymal nodules. Together, the occurrence of pulmonary nodules and pneumoconiosis (chronic inflammation of the lungs) creates a disorder called Caplan syndrome. Diffuse pulmonary fibrosis may occur because of immunologically mediated immune complex deposition. Rheumatoid nodules within the heart may cause deformities of the valves, particularly the aortic valve leaflets, and pericarditis. Lymphadenopathy of the nodes close to the affected joints may develop. Rheumatoid nodules within the spleen result in splenomegaly.

Another complication arises when these cysts rupture. This usually takes place when exercise or some other activity puts excessive pressure on the joint. Rupture releases inflammatory exudates into adjacent tissues, thereby spreading inflammation.

Other complications include the destruction of the tooth-like (odontoid) process of the second cervical vertebra. Sometimes cord compression can occur, particularly in patients with long-standing deforming RA. Such upper motor neuron signs as a positive Babinski reflex and muscle weakness may also develop. RA can also cause temporomandibular joint disease, which impairs chewing and causes earaches.

Did you know?

A study carried out by the State University of New York at Stony Brook, between October 1996 and December 1997, showed that RA patients who wrote about "the most stressful times in their lives" experienced significant reductions in disease activity within four months. Keeping a daily journal really can help relieve pain!

Chapter 2

Treatment

In addition to the conventional or alternative forms of treatment (see separately); patients with RA should sleep 10 to 12 hours out of each 24-hour period and maintain careful posture during this time. They should not use pillows or other devices that support the joints in a flexed position. They should use a firm mattress and only one pillow under the head. During periods of severe attacks, the patient may require continuous bed rest in order to allow the body's meagre natural defences against inflammation to work the best they can. However, even in acute phases, we balance rest with prescribed exercises.

The goal of physical therapy is to prevent and correct deformities, control pain, strengthen weakened muscles, and improve function. We may use applications of heat or to improve circulation, promote relaxation, and relieve pain. When used in conjunction with exercise, heat can allow more freedom of joint movement. We can use various forms of heat, including dry (heat lamp or hot water bottles), or moist (paraffin baths, whirlpools etc), ultrasound, and diathermy. Diathermy uses of high-frequency electrical currents to deliver moderate heat directly to the deeper tissues of the body. Exercise and therapy also keep the joints mobile. Surgery is the last resort in cases of severe joint damage.

Interviews

Here we will read about the opinions, and receive advice, from many specialists wanting to guide you along the path to better health. You will find advice from nutritionists, nurses and alternative therapists, all wanting to help you find your way through the maze of information available and make it more accessible to you.

Firstly, Don Lemmon (donlemmon.com), top Internet nutritionist and celebrity fitness trainer, author and TV personality, talked with me about his views on arthritis and nutrition.

Q: What should someone with RA do to ensure that they stay mobile?

A: I believe that if you have use of your arms, you should reach and stretch with them daily. If you can walk or sit, you should do at least freestyle squats. Aging, or illness, do not limit us. We limit ourselves by not doing things. Much like games, we get good, quit, go back, and see that we are not as good. But after a few tries, we improve again.

Q: Is there an exercise regime you'd recommend bearing in mind many arthritics must use wheelchairs or have limited mobility?

A: Yes, begin with stretching so the muscles get blood and nourishment, which leads to strengthening and more mobility, which allows for greater resistance and normal movement in time.

Q: What's the definition of good nutrition? What do our bodies need?

A: Protein, carbs, fats, water, and exercise for oxygen, sleep for healing and nothing processed, from a can, box or sweetened.

Q: What food groups would you recommend we eat on a daily basis to maintain a healthy system?
A: I recommend breaking the four food groups into twelve, as that allows greater flexibility and wider variety, while never confusing beans or nuts for proteins or thinking certain carbs are either bad or good.

Q: What makes up a balanced meal and how do we know we got it right?
A: Depends on what meal, what you do before or after the meal and the time of day. We all certainly have different tastes so we factor that in as well.

Q: Would a vegetarian lifestyle benefit an arthritic?
A: We have fangs, pointy teeth. We are meat eaters. I'm not big on eating foods people abuse before preparation, but there's a reason vegetarians like veggie burgers and meat-flavoured soy foods. The body craves meat.

Q: Many arthritics are overweight often due to inactivity. Can you offer a food plan that could benefit them and promote weight loss?
A: Not true, I sit on my duff 16 hours a day, I go weeks without exercise and I look great. People get fat because they eat like piglets. They scoff at the health food junkie and then look for excuses to keep doing what put them in their rut. It's food, folks. Eat right for a week without exercise and see if you do not lean out. You will!

Q: Many nutritionists recommend that someone with RA stay away from illuminative organs such as kidney, heart and liver, as they contain waste products that someone who is already ill would have problems dealing with. Do you agree?

A: I agree, but we still need in the contents of those organs, the components that heal us.

Q: Do you have any advice to someone suffering with Rheumatoid Arthritis?
A: Start eating right, begin stretching through the pain, see a good therapist, drink more water, kick the sugar, alcohol, cigarettes, hydrogenated oils, soda, etc. That alone will make you feel a decade younger again.

Following on from what Don told me, I contacted Jon Redshaw, (nutrition-zone.co.uk) and he told me about the necessity of a good diet when you have RA from a registered nutritionist's point of view:

"Nutrition makes up an essential ingredient in the treatment and management of Rheumatoid Arthritis with 40 percent of sufferers responding positively to therapy. We should use nutritional management of the disease alongside prescribed medication. Your nutritionist will look at a few key areas. The first area is food intolerances, which may trigger the disease. In RA, these are very diverse and due to this, the elimination diet tends to be very severe. Usually your nutritionist will use a "symptoms diary" prior to the elimination diet to establish what foods may trigger the disease. Removing certain foods from the diet has produced significant results with RA. Although the process can be tough, the results are always worth it.

"Once possible food triggers leave your diet, your nutritionist will then asses your general diet and immune system. Due to the inflammatory nature of RA, this will focus around altering your immune system to a more anti-inflammatory mode. We do this through dietary interventions and supplementation, usually to great effect. The nutritionist may also wish to supplement your antioxidant defence system, which mops up free radicals in the body. Because of the nature of RA, we likely cannot avoid supplements. Your nutritionist may also look at approaches such as the vegan diet, which shows very positive results with RA.

When choosing your nutritionist, you should check that he or she is suitably qualified, because anyone can call himself or herself a nutritionist. Qualified nutritionists register with the Nutrition Society and should have either Nutr or ANutr after their name. Nutritional therapists are recognised by The British Association of Nutritional

Therapists and have BANT after their name. You can check your nutritionist's accreditation at the organisations' Website. In fact, whatever country you live in, always check the nutritionist belongs to that country's nutrition society.

Did you know?

Cigarette smoking ranks as one of the highest risk factors identified to date for RA. The result comes after an 18-year analysis of 83,000 patients who took part in the trials run by the Nurse's Health Study, which ran from 1980-1998.

Pam Duff knows how diet can affect health first hand. Pam, a registered nurse, obtained certification in gerontology. She's spent more than thirty-six years studying nutrition in addition to her activities as a wife, mother, and grandmother. Her interest in nutrition began when her oldest son was diagnosed as hyperactive at the age of three. Doctors put him on Ritalin, but Pam soon took him off it because she did not like the results she saw. Since this occurred before the days of Dr. (first name?) Feingold and his diet theories, Pam had to figure out that diet changes were the key to helping her son, the rest of the family, as well as many other people at the time. After her forced, early retirement from the nursing profession due to a heart condition, Pam returned to diet as a means of healing. This led her to contribute the "health" section on the family's website (give address here).

I asked Pam to give us her thoughts on Rheumatoid Arthritis and the effects drugs have on the system. I found her research enlightening, not least because I'd been on most of the drug regimes she had described, and experienced many of their side effects, before I, too, turned to alternative methods of coping.

"As with cancer, people often mistakenly assume that arthritis presents the same symptoms and dysfunction in each person who has the disease. Such is not the case. Granted, there are many similarities, but generally, there are individual differences. Modern medicine often does not consider individuality. Instead, it tries to cover all bases with a one-size-fits-all pharmaceutical. Consequently, sufferers gain only marginal relief as these drugs cover up what really happens in the body. As consumers gain perception, they choose alternatives.

"As a retired registered nurse, I saw first hand just what drugs could do and what they cannot. Mostly, they cannot. They cannot cure the ailment nor can they not stop the myriad of side effects. Drugs of any description only mask symptoms. They do not permanently take care of a problem. When side effects occur, and they always occur, another drug has to take care of those. In the meantime, the original condition continues to grow. No drug on the market today cures anything! Drugs only to make you 'think' the problem has gone away.

There are over 100 different kinds of arthritis. They

include inflammatory and non-inflammatory, infectious and non-infectious, with varying symptoms and causes. The best guess anyone can make as to a commonality is that arthritis affects the joints. How then, with such a wide variety of processes taking place in individuals, can we expect to 'cure' all arthritis types with one simple pain pill?

Conventional doctors are more likely to prescribe an anti-inflammatory drug early in the disease. They believe that, as soon as the inflammation is suppressed, joints will not deteriorate but should improve, and patients will suffer fewer side effects if they receive treatment sooner rather than later. Rheumatologists believe that accurate diagnosis and appropriate intervention with drugs and physiotherapy in the early stage of the disease is crucial because the longer the inflammation lasts, the more damage occurs. However, we must stress that drugs may reduce inflammation, but they also take away warning symptoms (pain) and do nothing to reduce joint deterioration.

Despite the successful growth of alternative therapies for the treatment of arthritis, doctors and patients alike habitually treat the disease with drugs. This is understandable since most people will do anything to find quick relief. However, we pay a much greater price for that choice. The body can heal itself when given the proper tools —and drugs are definitely not proper tools. The following gives you an idea why:

Acetaminophen is an analgesic and antipyretic, which means it relieves pain and lowers fevers. We often use it instead of aspirin and it's sold under such trade names as Tylenol, Datril, and Liquiprin. As an arthritis treatment, we use it if we have pain but no inflammation, usually the case with osteoarthritis. However, when taken over a long period, acetaminophen can cause a significant decrease in liver function. It also causes many cases of kidney failure each year.

Aspirin (acetylsalicylic acid) is a common drug used to relieve pain and reduce fevers, but it has fallen into disfavor over recent years because of its association with the development of Reye's syndrome if taken during a viral infection. In the past, patients took this medicine for arthritic disorders, but not much any more. Taking aspirin will cause a reduction in vitamin C absorption, as well as a loss of iron and folic acid in the blood. It will also prolong bleeding time.

Corticosteroids (steroids for short) are hormones. The body produces some naturally, while others are manufactured synthetically. Those used in the treatment of arthritis come from, or are synthetic variants of, the natural corticosteroid hormones formed in the adrenal glands. When present in large quantities, they not only reduce inflammation, but they suppress immune responses, a supposed desirable effect for such autoimmune disorders as Rheumatoid Arthritis and other types of rheumatic diseases. However, a depressed immune system causes disease in the first place. Therefore, depressing the system even more allows other pathogens to enter the body, thereby increasing the risk of other diseases.

Corticosteroids wreak havoc with the body's nutritional status, decreasing the absorption of vitamin D and speeding up the excretion of zinc, potassium, and vitamin C. With the loss of such vital nutrients, the body deteriorates even further. More than three steroid shots per year can cause dangerous side effects in the central nervous system, endocrine system, cardiovascular system, and the eyes.

DMARDs (disease-modifying antirheumatic drugs) are given as treatment for Rheumatoid Arthritis, as well as such other types of rheumatic diseases as ankylosing spondylitis or psoriasis-linked arthritis. Health practitioners say DMARDs lower disease activity and inflammation, thereby reducing pain, swelling, and stiffness of joints. However, they have potentially more damaging side effects than NSAIDs. They act slowly, taking weeks or even months before the patient feels the full benefit. Because they are not analgesics, patients must take both, thus magnifying the risk of even more side effects.

NSAIDs (non-steroidal anti-inflammatory drugs) are most often prescribed for arthritis, and come under such names as aspirin, Advil, Aleve, Excedrin-IB, and Motrin. Doctors also use them as an alternative to such corticosteroids as cortisone and prednisone. Although they work on reduction of pain and inflammation, corticosteroids do have some nasty side effects. This led to the development of NSAIDs.

NSAIDs reduce inflammation in the joint linings by blocking the production of prostaglandins (hormone-like substances that cause the pain responses in the body). Prostaglandins also have other duties, including helping to regulate blood pressure, kidney function, and blood coagulation, as well as playing a role in the secretion of gastric acids. Anything that interferes with the "bad" actions of the prostaglandins will also hamper the "good" ones.

NSAIDs are either short acting (giving fewer than six hours of pain relief) or long-acting (bringing ten hours or more of relief). The body rapidly absorbs short-acting medications, thus they act acting quickly on symptoms. But the body also rapidly eliminates them, which helps prevent toxic accumulations. However, this also means the patient must take more of them. Long-acting medications are taken once, and then forgotten for the rest of the day. However, this also means they stay in the body longer, increasing the risk of toxic reactions. This is why doctors don't presecibe them for patients with kidney problems or for the elderly.

Taking high doses of NSAIDs, or taking them over a long period of time, can interfere with vital bodily activities and trigger such side effects as nausea, cramps, indigestion, diarrhoea, constipation, sensitivity to sunlight, nervousness, drowsiness, headaches, ulcers or stomach bleeding, sore throats or fevers (which may indicate bone marrow disorders), swelling of fingers, hands, feet and weight gain (which may indicate heart or kidney disorders), anaphylaxis (a potentially deadly allergic reaction), and high blood pressure (especially in those already having a problem with hypertension, dizziness, ringing in the ears, headaches, skin rashes, and depression).

Long-term use can also damage the stomach, and buffering the drug with an antacid is not effective in reducing this risk. Not only that, but antacids cause many other problems. Older adults, smokers, and those who consume alcohol are most at risk for stomach damage in the form of ulcers or gastrointestinal bleeding.

In addition, evidence shows that NSAIDs may inhibit the synthesis of proteoglycans – those important molecules that attract water to cartilage. Therefore, the medications we normally use to block pain may actually decrease the action of proteoglycans.

Chapter 3

Alternative Therapies and Supplements

In this section, we will look at alternative therapies and supplements available to the arthritic and that can either replace or compliment conventional medicine. Despite what doctors think, both can work together and treat the whole self rather than the symptoms themselves. At this present time the medical community does not recognise alternative therapies as beneficial, but as many people will testify, they not only benefit the patient but in some cases they successfully manage conditions that conventional medicine cannot.

Complementary Treatments

Complementary medicine believes that an accumulation of waste contributes to disease. Years of eating the wrong foods, not obtaining enough exercise, and living in a polluted environment tax the body earlier in life than before, causing disease more frequently and at a younger age.

Complementary therapies offer primarily a gentle approach. They are non-aggressive, non-invasive, and do not set up adverse reactions as can occur with conventional therapies. These treatments are designed to energize the whole body and to ease the pain and discomfort of the disease.

Conventional medicine relies mainly on such

pharmaceuticals as salicylates (especially aspirin), as well as non-steroidal and anti-inflammatory agents, anti-malarias, gold salts, and corticosteroids to override symptoms. However, this approach does not address the cause nor does it improve the overall general health of the body. Complementary medicine, on the other hand, takes a holistic approach, treating not only the disease, but also the health and well-being of the entire body by finding the cause and eliminating it. The following complementary therapies treat specifically arthritis.

Acupressure uses pressure on specific points of the body to stimulate them into moving along the *qi*, or life's force, which unclogs meridians that may cause a particular ailment. Using pressure points can greatly relieve the pain but may have to be undertaken at least two or three times a day in order to gain benefits.

- One such pressure point for pain in general is *Li4* (liver median), one of the most important points in acupressure and acupuncture therapies. It relieves headaches and other pain, relaxes tense muscles, and helps to balance the flow of energy between the upper and lower parts of the body. It's also used to clear excess heat from the body and to promote healthy functioning of the bowels. Find it in the middle of the fleshy mound in the webbing between the thumb and index finger. Use the thumb and index finger of the other hand; squeeze the centre of the webbing pressing toward the bone of the index finger. Hold one minute and repeat with the other hand.
- Another area is *Gb41* (gall bladder median). This is located on top of the foot in the channel between the little toe and the fourth toe, slightly less than halfway between the anklebone and the web margin between the

toes, but closer to the toes. The pain and discomfort of RA, plus the emotional response to that pain, can constrict the circulation of energy flow. This point helps restore that flow. Press with an index finger or middle finger, using firm pressure. Remember to start with light pressure, build up, hold, and gradually release.

⁂ *Gb34* is located at the lower border of the kneecap. Slide your finger off the shinbone below the knee toward the outside of the leg to a place where the two bones come together. Press in the soft tissue area between them using an index finger or both an index finger and middle finger together. This is a major pressure point for nourishing the tendons and joints. It also has a strong effect on promoting the smooth flow of life energy throughout the body. Obstruction of the smooth flow causes pain and discomfort. Disorders of the bone and cartilage relate to kidney energy. This is why, for OA (osteoarthritis), it is beneficial to strengthen kidney energy.

⁂ *K3* is considered the source point of the kidney meridian and the root of the "Yin and Yang" of the entire body. You will find it on the inside of the inner anklebone and the Achilles tendon on the back edge of the ankle. To locate, place your thumb on the bony prominence of the anklebone, on the inside area of the leg, and slide the thumb back towards the Achilles tendon. K3 lies in the depression about halfway between the anklebone and the back of the ankle. Press the thumb in this area, using medium to firm pressure for about a minute. Release slowly. Repeat on the other side.

Acupuncture uses specialized needles to stimulate painlessly the body's medians into removing any toxic buildup which causes disease. It is a deep tissue form of acupressure. Acupuncturists treat more patients with arthritis and back pain than any other complaint. Rheumatoid Arthritis responds extremely well to this traditional Chinese therapy. Dettox pads, or sap sheets also stimulate points on the feet.

Alexander technique was developed with the understanding that the way in which one uses his body affects how well it functions. This technique calls for improving postural habits, which can grow off-centred when pain affects a particular limb to the extent that it changes the overall body movement in order to accommodate that joint.

Aromatherapy, a centuries-long beauty and relaxation therapy, also offers medical benefits. Several recipes use essential oils in hot water, which are then applied to the painful joints. Many of these herbal oils help relieve pain and inflammation, though we can offer no guarantees. As with most therapies, what works for one may not for another. Pine, cypress, and cayenne make up the list of suggested oils. As arthritics can also suffer from stress, they can benefit from lavender and camomile oils an hour before bed used in an oil burner.

Biofeedback therapy uses sophisticated machinery to teach self-control over automatic and reflex-regulated body functions. The visual or auditory response of a highly sensitive machine allows the conscious or unconscious perception of physiological functions to be regulated, as that of the heart, skin temperature, and brain waves. The patient receives instant feedback on the state of his health. With biofeedback, people bring about their own physiological changes by re-educating the body. For the arthritic, the main benefit is the control or relief of pain, which helps to lessen the reliance on painkilling drugs.

Chiropractic is similar to osteopathy in that it alleviates the pain through the manipulation of the joint. The main difference between the two disciplines is that chiropractors use X-rays extensively to diagnose various problems while osteopaths rely on their knowledge of the human body to locate dysfunction and immobility. Chiropractors believe that X-rays make diagnosis more accurate and enables them to go straight to the problem. The arthritic sufferer needs to choose between the concern for using X-rays and the radiation from them, and how much the affected joint can be manipulated without undue pain.

Colour therapy comes from the view that colour affects not only moods and feelings but also total physical health and well-being. Since we know the colour of a room can affect one's mood, it should not be a shock that colour can also affect the immune system. The theory of colour therapy suggests that the body absorbs colour in the form of electromagnetic components of light and then produces its own aura of electro-magnetism. This aura gives off a pattern of vibration that a skilled colour therapist can discern. Red, for example, indicates anger, while dark shades of green mean envy (and thus the reason behind the infamous idiom "green with envy"). Disease manifests itself in the aura as a grey mass of accumulated energy. If the patient lets this go untreated, it will continue to manifest itself and turn into a physical symptom. When it reaches this stage, the colour therapist will have to disperse this mass of stagnant energy by reintroducing the colour frequency into both the physical body and the aura. The colours most used for arthritis are red, orange, gold, yellow, green, turquoise, blue, indigo, violet, and magenta.

Counselling is not so much an alternative answer to treating arthritis, as a support. Even conventional medicine recognizes the powerful link between the mind and the body and recommends some form of counselling to help cope with a disease process.

Dance therapy we recognise as a tremendous benefit, especially for those with a weakened immune system. Arthritic sufferers can profit by attending some form of dance class or dance exercise group. Music tends to unlock energy in the human body by stimulating, motivating, supporting, and balancing it. Dance helps to strengthen muscles and joints and regulates the breathing and circulation. Developed in 1929 by Heinrich Medau, a teacher of music and physical education in Berlin, the Medau movement formalises a natural system of dance. This derives from the structure of the body rather than by imposing any distortion or rigidity onto it. There are no jerky repetitions or overstretching. Another of the newest dance movement therapies comes from the theories of Rudolph Laban. Its design enables people to express their feelings while harmonizing both body and mind through the power of movement. Other types suitable for the arthritic and his/her personality also exist.

Exercise has long been thought of as aggravating or even causing osteoarthritis, and so many doctors advised against it. The natural tendency also leans in that direction–when an area hurts, stop using it! Exercise has many emotional and psychological benefits as well.

. Studies show it improves the mood because exercise releases endorphins, substances the brain secretes to help mask pain and bring about a feeling of euphoria. Exercise also helps decrease anger and hostility, reduce stress, and improve the memory and learning potential. Many of these stressors aggravate arthritic conditions. Today, we know that lack of exercise can devastate for the whole body, including the joints. In fact, a lack of exercise promotes the development of high blood pressure, obesity, diabetes, and heart disease.

A sedentary lifestyle ranks second only to smoking as the most common cause of disease and death in the United States alone. The United Kingdom ranks close behind. Even the simplest of exercises helps tremendously helpful by stimulating the cardiovascular system and thereby improving all body systems. A lack of exercise will also weaken bone structure, thereby increasing the risk of fractures as well as degeneration in general.

The following reasons show why exercise helps arthritics, in particular.

- Exercise encourages the flow of synovium fluid into and out of the cartilage. This fluid lubricates and nourishes cartilage, and its very presence can slow the progression of arthritis.
- Exercise strengthens the supporting structures -- muscles, tendons, and ligaments, as well as increasing the range of motion, shock absorption, and flexibility of the joints.
- Exercise improves overall physical capabilities, as well as improving emotional health.
- Exercise prevents joint deformities.
- Exercise reduces stress, thereby promoting relaxation and enhancing sleep.
- Exercise improves overall body composition by

promoting muscle strength and tone and decreasing fat.

* Exercise stimulates the immune system, thereby building a resistance to disease while building up a reserve capacity in the event of disease.

* Exercise improves sexual function, satisfaction, and body image.

* Exercise improves balance.

* Exercise helps preserve independence for a longer period.

* Exercise strengthens bones. Since bones are living matter, they change constantly. The osteoclasts continually tear down old bone cells, and osteoblasts continually build new ones. Weight-bearing and strength-training exercises increase bone density.

* The following exercise therapies are not too strenuous for the arthritic:

* Aerobics include brisk walking, jogging, or swimming. Patients should exercise for a minimum of thirty to forty-five minutes at least three times a week. Consistent moderate aerobic exercise over a longer period offers more benefits than strenuous exercise done in short burst.

* Brisk walking ranks as the very best aerobic exercise because the heart works at a safe rate, which promotes cardiovascular fitness. A regular walking program can enhance endurance, increase oxygen uptake, improve circulation and muscle tone, promote weight loss, and release toxins through perspiration. Walking also helps with emotional cleansing by reducing anxiety, stress, and depression.

* Pool exercises are excellent as the water acts as a giant cushion, absorbing the shock of movements and providing low-impact movement. Because water has more resistance than air, exercising in water causes the

leg muscles, heart, and lungs to work harder despite the slower speed. However, pool water can threaten asthmatics and those sensitive to chlorine.

⁂ Cycling, not a weight-bearing activity, puts less stress on the joints. Cycling can benefit us as much as running, increasing circulation and the flow of oxygen to the cells and helping to eliminate toxins. Stationary bicycles offer more environmental control and safety than outdoor cycling. The best stationary bikes exercise both the arms and the legs.

⁂ Chi kung and tai chi, two of the most popular martial arts disciplines, offer the same effectiveness as aerobic exercises in cleansing and detoxifying. Chi kung (qigong) is a Chinese term applied to many different forms of exercise that work with the chi (breath).

Kung means discipline, essentially "one who spends time practicing." Therefore, we can interpret chi kung to mean "the practice of proper breathing." It also provides motions to enhance and strengthen the body as a whole, which we use for treating chronic diseases. Tai chi is a series of continuous, slow, fluid, and graceful movements performed in a relaxed manner, with the knees slightly bent and the body in a straight, upright position. Described as "meditation in motion," tai chi involves a series of harmonious movements during which one focuses on the breath. When correctly performed, tai chi can stimulate circulation, detoxify, relax the joints, and encourage mental relaxation.

Herbal medicine seen as the mainstay of health since time began, ranked with "snake oil" within the last fifty years or so of the 1900s. However, it's once again regaining importance as an effective and safe treatment for most diseases. The blending of some herbs and water or oil for use internally and externally is both effective and soothing to the arthritic sufferer.

Herbs work quite differently from pharmaceutical drugs. Herbal anti-inflammatory preparations are not used as a means to suppress inflammation, which is a part of a healthy body response. Rather, these herbs help the body to overcome the problem, reducing inflammation naturally–unlike conventional anti-inflammatory drugs.

Herbs help restore balance and harmony to the whole body rather than simply treating symptoms. Because they use the whole plant rather than its isolated chemicals, the patient sees less risk of overdose or adverse side effects. However, we must still use herbs in a knowledgeable fashion because some herbs can harm us.

Meadowsweet and White Willow are the herbs most often prescribed for arthritis. They contain aspirin-like compounds and have a potent anti-inflammatory action. Meadowsweet contains aspirin-like substances that reduce swelling and pain, and also offers a diuretic and hepatic. Thus it confronts the acute complaint, cleans and eliminates, all while clearing the root of the inflammation, which lies in an accumulation of waste and toxins. Devil's claw also offers relief from arthritis.

For gout sufferers, celery seed stimulates the elimination of uric acid while the use of corn silk or horsetail strengthens the kidneys. Nettle improves circulation and helps the body get rid of excess harmful acids.

Homeopathy is widely known as a treatment that uses tinctures for various ailments, another holistic form of healing that treats the mind and body as one. Homeopathic remedies do not treat specific ailments but rather uniquely treat the individual complaint by taking into account the patient's state of mind, outlook, personality, and general behaviour, as well as the illness itself. *Rhus tox* or *toxicodendrum* (poison ivy) is the basic remedy for joints and recommended for the types of arthritis that improve with the application of heat but grow worse after sitting for long periods. Bryonia is useful for very painful joint conditions made worse by the least movement, which improve after rest and the application of cold compresses. Calc. phos. (Calcium phosphate) helps arthritis of the hands. Calc. carb. (calcarea carbonica, oyster shell) contains large quantities of calcium useful in the treatment of osteoarthritis. Ars. alb. (White arsenic) is potentially lethal in the wrong hands, but when used by the homeopathic practitioner, it can bring relief to those with symptoms that grow worse at night and improve with heat.

Hydrotherapy is based on the theory that when the body's immersed in water, weight-bearing joints suffer less strain. Water gives a feeling of comfort, relaxation, and lightness of being. Although some people have the luxury of going to a spa, You can also receive help at home. Dead Sea minerals, as well as those from other spas, are now available in health food stores for home use. These cannot, by law, claim to heal arthritis, but many sufferers find them extremely effective when added to their bathwater.

Massage offers a long-time history of therapeutic help. Most pain clinics today offer the therapy in one form or another. Many different kinds of massage work on various types of ailments. Those with arthritis require a gentle type, which a physical therapist can recommend.

Meditation, the ultimate "mind-over-matter" therapy, helps many but not all, arthritic sufferers. The practice of settling the mind through conscious effort has been used for thousands of years. Many arthritic patients advocate it because stress and tension seem to aggravate the disease. Since relaxation is never harmful, it's a decided benefit for any disease.

Naturopathy provides a common sense approach to health based on the body's own healing capabilities. It's principally made up of natural resources, including fresh air, sunlight, exercise, rest, good nutrition, hygiene, relaxation, and hydrotherapy. The approach involves a person taking charge of his own health, and its very simplicity makes this approach feasible. Naturopaths undergo a lengthy and extensive all-round education that involves not only the basics in medicine but also that of natural therapies, including nutrition and herbal medicine.

Nutritional counselling plays an integral part of all therapies and complementary medical practitioners use it most often. Certain foods aggravate arthritic diseases, and counselling along these lines will help, not only the pain, but in the progression of the disease. Supplements of glucosamine and chondroitin sulfates produce exciting results in reversing the effects of arthritis. Other supplements containing flavonoids, pancreatic enzymes, and bromelain have anti-inflammatory properties that reduce pain. Food allergies aggravate symptoms of arthritis, such as those from the nightshade family. Most medical professionals advise a dietary reduction or elimination in tea, coffee, alcohol, colas, refined sugars, wheat, red meat, and dairy productsin order to improve arthritic conditions.

Osteopathy uses expert manipulation to treat pain by correcting bone and joint problems. Mainstream medicine accepts this treatment, based on the belief that the spine is the source of good health. When the spine gets out of alignment, other physical problems develop. Osteopathy and chiropractic treat identical conditions using similar techniques, but differences exist. Chiropractics use X-rays extensively while osteopaths do not. Osteopaths also do more soft-tissue manipulation than chiropractics. In addition, they also mobilize joints by traction or articulation, putting the joints through a full range of passive movement, something not usually practiced by chiropractics. Osteopathy is more suitable for osteoarthritis but less so for Rheumatoid Arthritis.

Psychotherapy, a "talking cure," is divided into three types: supportive, exploratory, and specialized. Supportive is the simplest and least intrusive with the client simply talking about personal problems and developing an atmosphere of trust and confidentiality. Exploratory therapy encourages the client to explore the problem rather than merely voicing it. The therapist will periodically intervene to point out inconsistencies, evasions, and neglected aspects of an issue, to help the person recognize causes and solutions to a problem. Specialized therapy involves behavioural psychotherapy, cognitive therapy, psychoanalysis, gestalt, psychodrama, and many other forms of therapies involving specialized intervention. The form most suitable for the arthritic is cognitive, which we can loosely as "positive thinking," likely one of the most powerful tools in fighting chronic pain and for coping with disability and immobility.

Reflexology is becoming more popular as a means to boost energy levels, promote a sense of well-being, and alleviate pain. Its foundational beliefs compare similarly to that of acupressure and acupuncture in that the life force (qi or chi) flows through the body along energy channels. However, in reflexology, the terminal points of the energy channels lie in the feet and hands while in acupuncture, they lie all over the body. Tension or congestion in any part of the body is mirrored in the corresponding reflex areas on the feet and hands. By applying controlled pressure to these areas in a precise and systematic way, the body can better achieve its own natural state of good health. One of the underlying theories holds that our ancestors walked and ran virtually barefoot over uneven ground, which constantly massaged and stimulated the nerve endings and reflex areas. Today, we spend too much time sitting. When walking, we should make sure we have well-cushioned shoes. Wearing high heels alters the joints of the feet all the way up the spine. This puts added strain on some areas while failing to stimulate others. Before long, waste products build up and the body does not eliminate them. Disease results. While reflexology cannot cure arthritis, it can help alleviate the pain and raise energy levels.

Relaxation therapy will not yield positive results in a day or even a week, but must be practiced for many weeks before the patient feels relief from pain. Holding stress and tension within the body for long periods sets it up for many adverse physical reactions. By learning specific breathing techniques and listening to calming music, a person will begin to relax and, in time, see his pain decrease and his overall physical and mental health improve.

Self-hypnosis is a form of deep relaxation as opposed to a trance-like state. The point of a deeply relaxed state lies in the person giving instructions to himself that the mind and body will obey. This method has proven somewhat successful in reducing chronic pain not alleviated by medication or surgery.

Shiatsu, a Japanese word, literally means "finger pressure." However, the shiatsu practitioner not only uses fingers but also hands, thumbs, elbows, and even knees or feet to achieve the desired depth and strength of massage. The pressure provided should produce a sensation somewhere between pain and pleasure. The system bears some similarities to acupressure as both are based on pressure points along meridian lines associated with the function of vital organs.

As in acupuncture, the shiatsu therapist will take the six pulses at each wrist. Each is associated with a vital organ in the body and by taking the pulses, the practitioner can diagnose and treat many different conditions. Arthritis sufferers may also benefit from a related technique known as "do-in," literally translated to mean "self-stimulation." This is a form of self-acupressure of muscles and points, as well as movement, stretching, and breathing exercises.

T'ai chi (or t'ai qi) increases oxygen flow to the blood and the joints of the body, especially the knees, alleviating the pain of inflammatory diseases. Relief from pain is an important concern for the arthritis sufferer, but only one of t'ai chi's benefits. Only twenty-four movements comprise t'ai chi, which , making it easier to adopt, helping to restore balance to the mind and body.

Visualization, a therapy developed in the 1960s by cancer specialists Carl and Stephanie Simonton, often helps in shrinking cancer cells. Their success transferred over into healing other diseases, including arthritis. By picturing the painful and swollen joints as whole and strong again, many sufferers found that they reversed their condition. Once again, this works for some but not others and depends on the individual personality.

Yoga combines postures and breathing with meditation to enable energy to travel throughout the body. This ancient system of breathing movements and postures not only brings tranquillity of body and mind but also enhances the flexibility of the spine, releases muscular tension, and increases the circulation to the organs and glands.

Yoga takes many different forms of yoga, but each has its own particular emphasis. For example, Hatha yoga concentrates on postures and movements that encourage the body to stretch and tone. Kundalini yoga concentrates on the spinal column, strengthening and balancing the nervous system.

Pranayama yoga focuses on breathing, strengthening, and balancing the respiratory system. Yoga can realign the spine or even prevent spinal misalignments. It reverses the effects of gravity's downward pull on the vital organs and glands in the body. Such inversion exercises as the shoulder stand increase the blood supply to organs and glands. Other postures stimulate the kidneys, liver, stomach, colon, and pancreas to promote cleansing and purification.

However, the arthritic should use the following positions to start with before attempting moves more strenuous. All movements depend on the range of motion for each joint.

- Supported leg raises: These provide a gentle stretch, ideal for relieving stiffness. Lie on your back and stretch your legs up against a wall. Stretch your arms above your head and keep the spine stretched. Hold for as long as comfortable.

- Corpse pose: This aids in complete relaxation of the mind and body. Lie on your back with your legs and arms straight but not tense. Rest your head on a folded towel or blanket. Take a few deep gentle breaths, and then breathe slowly and evenly. Stay in this position for at least 15 minutes.

⁕ Supported corpse pose: This particularly rests the back. Lie on your back with your head resting on a folded towel. Support your legs, bent at the knees, on a level chair or stool. Breathe evenly, and rest in this position for several minutes.

⁕ Seated pose: Sit with your legs out straight in front of you and your feet together. Support yourself with your hands and arch your spine.

⁕ Raised arms: Stand in a relaxed position with your feet together, knees slightly bent, and hands at your sides. With your shoulders relaxed, raise your arms above your head as you breathe in. Hold for as long as comfortable.

⁕ Basic standing posture: Keep a relaxed stance and breathe into the abdomen. Let the shoulders relax. Bring the neck, back, and hips forward to maintain a straight spine. Centre your weight on the balls of your feet.

About Audio Tapes for Healing

Ellen Gordon Knapp talked to me about her healing tapes. They harness the bodies' natural ability to self-heal and can promote great results. If you use these tapes, they will help you concentrate and float away from your pain promoting relief. If nothing else, you will feel stress free during use and that alone is worth it. Ellen said:

"I created Audiotapes for Healing out of a personal need for tools to help me relax when I feel overwhelmed or discouraged by the stress of having arthritis."

"The basic Relaxation and Healing tape and CD addresses the chronic stress of chronic illness, such as arthritis. Stress often makes arthritis symptoms worse, triggering flare-ups, weakening immune function and interfering with the ability to experience pleasure in everyday life."

The Basic Relaxation and Healing tape or CD:

Part 1 guides you to relax each part of your body. As you follow the directions, you will discover that you can use your mind to relax your body.

Part 2 guides you to create an imaginary healing sanctuary just for you. In this sanctuary, you feel protected and nurtured. You're free to do whatever it takes for you to heal. Once you feel relaxed, nurtured, and safe, the rest of the tape/CD guides you to see yourself healing.

Part 3 guides you to imagine healing energy filling your body. Not only is this a wonderful, healing image, but once you're accustomed to working with it, you have a valuable tool. With practice, you can replace gloomy thoughts with the thoughts of hope and healing that you hear on the tape.

Part 4 guides you to see yourself healed. This sends messages of health to your unconscious mind and to your body. Evidence shows that when you focus on images of a healthy self, your body listens and responds.

Listening to this tape at times of stress gives an effect of immediately calming you. For 25 minutes, mind and body live in a world of peace. Use it at bedtime for peaceful sleeping. Take a break in the middle of a stressful day and eliminate or lower your feelings of tension and anxiety.

After listening to the Relaxation and Healing tape or CD for several weeks, anytime you feel stressed you can use the techniques that you practised each time you listened to your tape and relaxed.

For example, while sitting in traffic, you can go through your body, asking each part to relax. You can imagine yourself in a beautiful vacation spot. You can picture healing energy filling your body. When you first listen to the tapes or CDs, you need the soothing voice of an expert to guide you through the steps to relax.

After several weeks of relaxing while listening to your tape or CD, you will begin to develop an ability to do this in any location.

Living with illness can create a cycle of stress. Having arthritis can cause you to feel stressed and living with stress can make the arthritis worse. Stress can suppress immune function, increase inflammation, increase susceptibility to infection and just take the joy out of living. All of the tapes and CDs reduce stress and increase relaxation. Relaxation and healing and the affirmation tapes and CDs replace negative thoughts with hopeful, nurturing thoughts.

Affirmation tapes and CDs for Pain, Surgery, Illness, Anxiety and Low Self-Esteem, a Healthy Lifestyle.

Affirmations are statements about good and positive elements in your life. The affirmations on my affirmations tapes and CDs counteract the negative, worrisome thoughts that crop up when we worry about our health.

The depression that sometimes accompanies arthritis can lead us to exaggerate the problems and ignore everything good about our life and ourselves. This makes the illness worse. We will have better health and happiness by dealing with our problems and then quickly putting our attention on what's good and hopeful.

Part one of each of the affirmation tapes and CDs has the Relaxation and Healing I describe above. It's easier to believe and accept new and positive ideas when you feel relaxed.

The affirmations are on side two of the tapes and track two of the CDs. This way you can listen to the affirmations after you're already relaxed. Another option is to listen to the affirmations by themselves at times when it's unsafe to listen to the relaxation part. For example, you can listen to the affirmations when you're working around the house or driving a car.

Sample affirmations from the Pain tape and CD:

- I am not the pain in my body.
- I am more than pain.
- I am able to observe the ways that my attachment to pain ebbs and flows.
- I have a life, and an awareness separate from pain.
- I ask God to help me relax around the pain.
- There are people in my life who care about me. As I receive their love, the pain lessens. I am not alone.

Sample affirmations from the Surgery tape and CD:

- Healing energy flows through my body.
- Loving friends and family surround me. Their love and good wishes help me to get well.
- During my surgery, I see myself surrounded by the healing energy generated by the prayers and good wishes of my family and friends.
- The entire hospital is filled with loving energy from the prayers of my family and friends.
- God is with my doctors and me during my surgery.
- Deep within me is the power to heal myself. I let go of concern, as I trust this healing power.
- I trust my doctors. I trust my body's innate ability to heal. I trust in the support of a loving universe

Sample affirmations from "A Healthy Lifestyle" tape and CD.

These affirmations help if you want to use diet and exercise as part of your healing protocol. Instead of complaining about the foods you give up, you focus on the benefits of healthy living.

- I want to live a healthy life. I commit to nurturing my body and my mind.
- I nurture myself with good habits of healthy living.
- I love my life and I appreciate my body.
- I enjoy eating well-prepared nourishing food.
- My food supports me. My food nourishes me and keeps me healthy.
- I exercise every day.
- When I exercise, I feel alive. I feel my body strengthening.
- When my resolve falters, I am willing to ask for help. I ask for help when I need it.
- I am not alone.

Sample affirmations from the Anxiety and Low Self-Esteem tape and CD:

- My body is relaxing. I am relaxing.
- I am calm. I am clear. I am focused.
- Whenever I feel myself getting anxious, I become quiet; I focus on my breath;
- I breathe in; I breathe out; and I remind myself that I am doing a good job.
- Every one of my problems has a solution.
- It is okay to ask for help.
- I am present in my life and I am functioning in this moment.

Sample affirmations from the Healing from Illness tape and CD:

- I want to be healed.
- I have a strong immune system.
- My treatment is working with my immune system to eliminate illness.
- My immune system is strong and healthy.
- Every day I feel stronger than the day before.
- Inflammation is leaving my body.
- Toxins are leaving my body.
- Healing energy flows through me. .
- I ask God to help me heal.
- I ask God to help me know I am okay just as I am.
- I feel my heart opening to the love of all who care for me

About the Breathing Meditation

With the breathing meditation, you practice focusing. You practice quieting the mind's usual flow of thoughts by putting all your attention on a single object: your breath. A mind full of racing thoughts creates stress and fatigue. Because the breathing meditation practice quiets those thoughts, it relaxes and energizes.

In the breathing meditation, you focus attention on your physical sensations as you breathe. With each breath, you observe the feeling of the air moving in and out of your lungs.

Chronically stressed people typically hold their breath or breathe very shallowly. When they inhale, air typically fills only the top third of the lungs. Many exercises correct shallow breathing habits; I count the breathing meditation as my favourite.

The entire exercise involves spending a specific amount of time doing nothing but noticing your breath and noticing how your body feels as the air moves in and out of your body. You notice your breath, but you do not try to control it. When you begin, you will probably notice that on your inhalation, you feel only the air filling the top portion of your lungs. However, as you observe your breath *without controlling it*, your breath will go deeper and deeper with each inhalation until finally, air fills most of your lungs. When you decide not to control your breathing, it naturally goes deeper. This exercise requires no other effort.

You do not need a tape or CD to do this exercise of paying attention to your breath. However, when most people first begin to meditate, they find that the mind behaves like a spoiled child. It does not want to cooperate. You say to yourself, I'm going to focus on my breathing. You begin, but after a minute, you realize you're thinking about something else. Therefore, the Breathing Meditation tape acts as a coach. The tape contains little dialogue, because listening to dialogue distracts you from focusing on your breath. However, in case your mind has wandered, every 30 seconds a short reminder returns your focus to observing your breath.

Music therapist Kerry Lee plays the background music for Relaxation and Healing and the affirmation tapes and CD on the lyre. Ocean waves make up the background for the meditation tape and CD.

Relaxation and Healing tape and CD lasts 25 minutes. Relaxation and Healing with one of the affirmation tapes and CDs lasts approximately 50 minutes.

The Breathing Meditation takes 15 minutes. The Body Awareness Meditation goes for 35 minutes. You can find these types of tapes online and in stores.

Supplements

I have tried CMO, cerasomal-cis-9-cetyl myristoleate, several times over the past few years with amazing results. As I recovered from a total knee replacement operation due to Rheumatoid Arthritis, the disease started in my ankle. It was Catch-22. They cured the knee but the illness migrated to the ankle. I fell into the blackness of self-pity and cried a lot of the time. My husband, distressed at this, did his own research on the Internet. He found David Harrison's website (cmo.inuk.com) and ordered two bottles. I did not find the diet fun, as I love my carbonated drinks and coffee, but I soon adapted and within a few days, I started to notice the pain ebbing away and my ankle loosening up again. At first I felt sceptical. After all, how could anything made from a meat derivative work? However, it did. I now firmly believe in CMO and every time I feel my illness flaring up, I order more. Within a few days I feel better again. This experience prompted me to contact *David Harrison of 'The CMO Company'* on your behalf and ask him about CMO. David supplied the following information to answer questions on CMO.

What is CMO?

Cerasomal-cis-9-cetyl myristoleate (CMO) pronounced ***sera-somal-cis-9-see-tul-meer-is-toll-ee-ate*** derives from beef tallow from BSE-free herds in the USA. It's a natural immunomoderator, trials offer proof that it stops the arthritic process in up to 90 percent of people who take it.

What conditions does CMO help?

CMO helps all forms of arthritis, except gout, but in particular osteoarthritis and Rheumatoid Arthritis, no matter how bad your symptoms get. According to anecdotal reports, CMO's helped other autoimmune diseases, although research into these types of diseases continues.

How does CMO work?

Studies show that arthritis is an autoimmune disease. This means that the body mistakenly identifies its own tissues as foreign and mounts an attack on them. We've known for a long time that Rheumatoid Arthritis results from this faulty immune response, but only recently did we find a similar cause for osteoarthritis.

We believe CMO works by reprogramming the faulty immune system so that it no longer views its own tissues as foreign and stops attacking them. Because CMO treats the cause of the arthritis, rheumatoid or osteo, and stops the arthritic process, the treatment rarely needs repeating. This makes it very different from other products on the market, which need to be taken regularly to maintain the benefits.

Does CMO stop my immune system from working?

CMO is not an immunosuppressant, nor an immunostimulant or a pharmaceutical. It comes from naturally substances and ranks at the highest safety level attainable by certified independent laboratory testing.

Unlike immunosuppressants, CMO does not leave the body vulnerable to attack by disease-causing agents. Neither does it inhibit the body's resistance to tumour formation, as do the dangerous new tumour necrosis factor (TNF) suppressants of some new drugs.

How was CMO discovered?

In 1971, a researcher at the National Institutes of Health, first discovered the predecessor of CMO capsules, cetyl myristoleate. No one agreed to find the researcher's project, so he slowly carried on at his own expense. Eventually, he discovered that when he injected this substance near the joints of lab animals, it brought amazing results, stopping the arthritis process in its tracks. Many years later, he experienced the same benefit on his own body. After his doctor could provide no further relief through conventional medicine, he successfully injected himself with cetyl myristoleate for the arthritis in his knees. The beneficial results so amazed his doctor that he urged his patient to publish a report.

In March of 1994, The Journal of Pharmaceutical Sciences published that report about injectable cetyl myristoleate.. In the report, the researcher expressed his hope that others would conduct studies, "particularly, more extensive tests of cetyl myristoleate analogues." A digestible form of CMO would allow arthritis sufferers to self-administer the treatment.

In late 1994, the International Immunological Centre of The San Diego Clinic research staff did exactly what that researcher had hoped. They developed an orally administered nutritional supplement. This dietary supplement is an analogue called CMO, a trade name for cerasomal-cis-9-cetylmyristoleate. The San Diego Clinic did the first clinical study on CMO, which demonstrated the substance as an outstanding product in the treatment of arthritis.

In December 1995, Nevada introduced CMO to the medical community at the National Medical Conference on Aging. Five doctors afflicted with a variety of conditions tried CMO. All five doctors responded well within three days. CMO starred at the conference, resulting ultimately in hundreds of doctors using it for their patients.

In February 1996, after successful reports from the medical community, the public could get CMO. Its beneficial effects have inspired many books about the subject.

Do I have to stick to a very rigid diet while taking CMO?

Originally, Dr. FIRST NAME Sands recommended a very restrictive diet while taking CMO, but over the years of research, he found that most patients could eat a relatively normal diet and still get good results. The patient must keep to foods and drinks that do not stress the liver or immune system. The following guidelines appear to work very well for the majority of patients:

Diet restrictions

For best results the patient must avoid the following while taking CMO and for two weeks after finishing all of the capsules. These substances stress the immune system, overload the liver, and reduce the effectiveness of CMO. You may return to your usual eating pattern after this time.

- Alcohol (beer, wine, cider, spirits)
- Products containing caffeine (coffee, tea, chocolate, colas, stimulant drinks, etc.) A limited amount, 1 cup, of any decaffeinated beverage each day is okay.
- Any foods that you know, from experience, may upset your body. Many people have found that "nightshade" vegetables such as potatoes, aubergine, peppers and tomatoes adversely affect their joint health.
- Laxatives, which may encourage elimination of CMO before absorption.
- Sweets. Sugar, in quantity, suppresses immunity.

Dr. Sands originally advised against the consumption of all grains. His later research suggested that most people did not need to do this. If you wish to play safe, you could cut out all wheat products while consuming CMO.

So what can I eat while taking CMO?

The simple answer: near enough anything!

Diet recommendations

You may eat the following while taking CMO.

* All lean meats of chicken, lamb, pork and especially beef – regular beefeaters often respond faster because their bodies create plenty of the exact natural enzymes needed to digest beef products and, therefore, CMO
* All fish–especially sardines, salmon, fresh tuna, mackerel, trout (all high in Omega 3 fats). If you do not enjoy eating fish, take extra Omega 3 supplements.
* All fruits, vegetables, unsalted nuts (except those known or suspected to upset you)
* Dairy products, in moderation, if you're in the habit of consuming them and they agree with you.
* High-quality protein, particularly soy and whey products, if you're vegetarian.
* A top-quality vitamin/mineral supplement daily plus Omega 3 capsules.

Also, drink at least eight half-pint glasses of plain water each day. We cannot overstate the importance of this recommendation.

How long will the benefits last?

A single CMO course usually lasts forever without any need to repeat. It treats the cause of the disease, not just the symptoms. If something subsequently triggers the immune system to attack the joints, then you might require a repeat dose, but we have patients who took CMO 10 years ago and still benefit from the single course.

Does CMO work for everyone?

We have found that about 90 percent of arthritis sufferers get good results. Most require only one bottle of CMO, but occasionally some need a second bottle, especially if they've taken steroids or other drugs which affect the immune system or liver.

Do I need more than one bottle of CMO?

Most of our patients find they only require one bottle of CMO to get rid of their arthritis. We generally advise that if you received absolutely no benefit from one bottle of CMO then, you probably won't gain relief by taking more. However, if you have received even marginal improvement from your arthritic symptoms from one bottle, we recommend a further course. People with poor liver or digestive systems may require more than one bottle of CMO.

If CMO is so terrific, why haven't I heard about it and why doesn't my doctor recommend it?

Doctors only slowly recognize and understand natural products. Despite huge amounts of research proving that CMO benefits Rheumatoid and osteoarthritis sufferers, the United States' Food and Drug Association guidelines and the United Kingrom's MHRA guidelines only allows marketing of CMO as a joint supplement. Thus it must compete with hundreds of products marketed the same way. Understanding of the extraordinary benefits is limited by prohibitions of expounding more on labels and web pages. To date, funding is unavaialable to allow the expensive testing required to obtain a medicines licence. Word of mouth is the best advertising for CMO and most other natural products.

Most doctors obtain their postgraduate information from medical literature sponsored by the large drug companies. Natural remedies, which may affect the profits of these companies, therefore seldom get published. The health service treatment protocols seldom include natural products and few doctors have training or personal experience with natural products' benefits or use. Doctors can only prescribe licensed medicines. It costs millions of pounds to obtain a license. CMO, a natural product, cannot be patented. The manufacturers of CMO, at least four of them in the United States, likely will not pay the money to get the product licensed, because that would allow other companies to sell their CMO under the same license.

Why doesn't CMO work equally well for everyone?

We do not know why CMO does not work for 10 percent of the population, but we know of six situations, other than this normal biological uniqueness, that hinder its effectiveness:

1.**Failure to follow the recommended dietary plan**. Before trying a second or third bottle, non responders might try eliminating possible food trigger factors like wheat, corn, and other grains. Eliminating dairy products may help.

2.**Impaired liver function**—even slight impairment not detectable by common lab tests. Usually the result of current or previous infection (hepatitis, Epstein-Barr, mycoplasma, chlamydia, etc.) or previous or current substance use (alcohol, steroids, methotrexate, excessive paracetamol, anti-inflammatory or analgesics, etc.). One possible solution: take the herb milk thistle (Silymarin) for 30 days before beginning or continuing CMO.

3. **Continuing underlying low-grade systemic or localized infections** caused by viral agents (usually herpes simplex, HHV-6, Epstein–Barr, etc.), or bacteria (usually staph, strep, chlamydia or mycoplasms).

4. A faulty digestive system incapable of absorbing CMO as a result of impaired fat/protein digestion, impacted waste buildup in the intestines, frequent loose stools or other digestive problems. Adding an enzyme product containing lipase, protease and amylase to one's diet might help.

5. **Continued exposure to ambient sensitivity factors** in the home, workplace or geographical area (insecticides, pollen, dust, plastics, other chemicals, insulation, carpets, petroleum, vapors, etc.).

6. Unrecognised or under-treated hypothyroidism. (See below)

Thyroid problems

We have repeatedly noticed a correlation between people with low body temperature and/or other symptoms of low thyroid function and minimal or no response to CMO. (Go to www.wilsonssyndrome.com for a list of low thyroid symptoms.) According to Denis Wilson, M.D., and other health professionals, a body temperature consistently below normal, along with other symptoms, may indicate of an underactive thyroid or under- treated or mistreated thyroid condition. If you take thyroid medication or your doctor has told you your thyroid blood tests are normal, and you still have symptoms of sluggish thyroid function, CMO may not benefit you. The thyroid gland secretes a hormone, thyroxin, essential for thymus activity. If the thyroid fails to function well, either naturally or with the help of effective hormone treatment, CMO is often ineffective.

Can I test for myself for correct thyroid function?

The simplest test to see if your thyroid functions correctly is to take your temperature three times over a 24 hour period. If it shows up consistently half a degree or more below normal, then you may have low thyroid function.

You could attribute this to an iodine deficiency as your body needs iodine in order to manufacture thyroxine, the thyroid hormone.

Luckily, an excellent home test checks your own iodine levels. Simply take a cotton bud, dip it into a 2% tincture of iodine (available at the pharmacist or supermarket), and paint an area the size of a ten-cent coin on your thigh or abdomen, leaving a yellowish stain that should disappear in about 24 hours if your iodine levels are normal. If the stain disappears in less than 24 hours, it indicates a possible deficiency in iodine. If so, it may be worth taking Kelp, excellent iodine supplement.

Some people who did not initially respond to CMO did so after increasing their iodine intake by taking kelp. You can get it in capsule form from your health food shop or pharmacist. Ask your health care provider to test your iodine level and make a supplement recommendation if he feels it's appropriate. Some cases of low thyroid activity come from excessive iodine in the system. Therefore you should seek professional medical advice.

Also, you should not change the amount of any prescription drug you take without consulting your prescribing doctor.

How do I know if a company is selling "genuine CMO"?

Capsules should contain 385 mg of CMO and for best results should contain digestive enzymes. You can find several similarly potent versions. Some contain digestive enzymes and other additional ingredients. Different private brand labels market these products.There is simply no one authentic, true CMO, as some marketers insist. Most frequently CMO distributors hear, "How do I know this is the REAL CMO?" If the product contains at least 385 mg per capsule of cerasomal-cis-9-cetyl myristoleate, (not cetyl myristoleate) and comes with a money-back guarantee that allows you to try the product and get a refund if it does not help you, then it's likely genuine. If a company's selling substandard CMO (usually in the form of cetyl myristoleate rather than the correct form cerasomal cis 9 Cetyl myristoleate), they are unlikely to give you any guarantee.

Can you recommend a company that sells genuine CMO?

The only company in the United Kingdom and Europe to give a money-back guarantee is The CMO Company. David Harrison, a registered osteopath, runs this company from his busy osteopathic clinic in Somerset, UK. For further information, and to place orders, you can reach him at the address in the resources section:

The San Diego Clinic recommends the company as suppliers of genuine CMO, and it gives a full money-back guarantee on its product. The company gives a free advice and backup service, and the capsules contain the correct dosage of CMO and digestive enzymes to give optimum results.

Green Lipped Mussels and Arthritis

I spoke to Lesley Cutts (goodnessdirect.co.uk) about Green Lipped Mussels and their benefits to the RA sufferer and she told me how they could help. Again I took this for a while and did notice a significant improvement in my illness. However, they don't suit everyone and you should take care and read the label before trying them.

American researchers looking for treatments for cancer from the sea, back in the '60s, made the original discovery that Green Lipped Mussel may help arthritis. The New Zealand Green Lipped Mussel made the list of shellfish undergoing study. During this research, they coincidentally found that Green Lipped Mussel has anti-inflammatory properties, unique to this particular mussel. Hence the connection with arthritis.

Arthritis is essentially inflammation in a joint. We can list more than two hundred types of arthritis, but two types are most common: inflammation of a joint for an unknown cause (as in Rheumatoid Arthritis) and wear and tear arthritis where the joint wears out and rough, thickened areas develop in place of the smooth cartilage which enables easy, smooth movement of the joint (as in osteoarthritis).

Clinical trials on Green Lipped Mussel extract have shown beneficial results for patients suffering from both types of arthritis.

We commonly treat the pain and stiffness associated with arthritis with anti-inflammatory drugs, one of the most common side effects of which are gastric disorders, or the irritation of the stomach and upsetting of the digestive system.

However, Green Lipped Mussel offers very few side effects, mostly mild gastro-intestinal distress. This particularly makes a difference for elderly patients who may develop a gastric or duodenal ulcer during treatment with conventional non-steroidal anti-inflammatory drugs. However, we've seen allergic reactions; people who suffer from an allergy to shellfish or gelatine should not use the product.

Anti-inflammatory properties of Green Lipped Mussel

Because of the discovery in the '60s, research on the anti-inflammatory properties of green lipped mussels began in 1973 and still continues. Studies so far indicate that it's associated with a glycoprotein consisting of glycogen, a complex form of sugar tied up with one of the proteins. Glycogen's a sugar stored in the mussel's muscle. It's found in all animals and is utilised in energy production.

Glycogen complex suppresses some swelling.
An antihistamine substance isolated from the New Zealand Green Lipped Mussel extract also shows a preventive action against arthritis.

Conclusion

People in more than twenty countries take Green Lipped Mussel as a food supplement, mainly to help maintain mobility of the joints. The potential benefits may take effect gradually. We recommend and a regular course over several months. One of the major benefits demonstrated by scientific studies is the extract's gentleness on the stomach. You can take it safely at the same time as most prescribed medication or medicines. NB Seatone contains natural sea salts and should those suffering from, or taking medication for, high blood pressure, should not take it.

Tuna Capsules

Jeanette Bradley of Wellcene (wellcene.co.uk) talked to me about their tuna capsules, and after trying them for myself, I believe they offer help, as I feel much better and more awake than I have for a long time. Tiredness became a daily companion.

Arthritis is a common chronic systemic inflammatory disease that results in progressive disability. Inflammation of the synovium primarily characterises it. As the disease progresses, the patient suffers destruction of cartilage and bone. Without a cure, we try to manage it to relieve pain and improve or maintaining joint function.

Fish oils containing n-3 fatty acids (Omega 3 fatty

acids) reportedly to decrease pain and stiffness in arthritis. The n-3 fatty acids found in fish oil, namely Eicosapentaenoic acid (EPA) and Docosahexaenoic acid (DHA), can suppress the production of inflammatory eicosanoids and cytokines; and suppress the production of cartilage degradative enzymes.

Tuna capsules contain oil from the body of the fish and not the eliminative organ as in Cod Liver Oil capsules. Therefore, they are a great alternative to anyone wanting to cut these out of the diet and are beneficial to the arthritic in maintaining joint mobility.

What can help?

Throughout my research, I have found that we can reverse or prevent the vast majority of arthritic conditions through diet and the use of a selected number of supplements. Of course, we can't ignore exercise. Exercise keeps the joints limber and also relieves the stressors that trigger worsening arthritic symptoms.

Again, the kind of exercise depends on the person and what he/she feels comfortable doing. You should not dance if you hate the activity and much prefer to take long walks. This is another example of the importance of treating the individual. Without a change in diet though, arthritic sufferers simply will not feel well enough to participate in any activity. Today, doctors take diet more seriously, as mounting evidence proves that nutrition plays an important role in any disease, including arthritis, especially Rheumatoid Arthritis.

Arthritis and food sensitivities have a long history, and the disease can result from ignoring such occurrences. For example, many arthritic sufferers feel worse first thing in the morning. Generally, we believe that the immobility of sleep brings on stiffness, and that might contribute. People believe that morning stiffness results from not eating the foods to which the individual is sensitive for a longer period, as happens after a nighttime of rest. These people also feel worse if they happen to miss breakfast, which normally contains at least one of the offending foods. This may sound contradictory, but studies show that the body craves foods which create sensitivity or allergy.

For the sensitive individual, food proteins can cause much the same reaction as a grass, mould, pollen, peanuts, or any other allergen. When an allergen enters the body, it provokes an immune response, which releases inflammatory mediators, causing hypersensitive reactions. When food passes into the gastro-intestinal tract and acts like an allergen, the immune system responds by producing an antibody that binds to the food in an attempt to neutralize it. One specific immunoglobulin that is supposed to help with the regulation and neutralization of these food allergens is IgA. However, the production of IgA is much lower in individuals with Rheumatoid Arthritis than in unaffected people or even those with non-inflammatory arthritis. Research shows that some with Rheumatoid Arthritis abnormally digest and absorb wheat and dairy products. Their gastro-intestinal tracts appear to be more permeable to these foods making them act as antigens or allergens.

Arachidonic acid looks like the main food culprit when it comes to producing inflammation. It is found almost entirely in animal products and saturated fats. Animal products increase the production of the inflammatory chemicals, prostaglandins, and leukotrienes. Not only does arachidonic acid produce prostaglandins responsible for inflammation but also the kind that produces platelet stickiness that leads to hardening of the arteries, heart disease, and strokes.

Studies show that if we remove, or at the very least, limit, animal products in the diet, symptoms of arthritis begin to disappear. When the consumption of these foods increases, we see a corresponding increase in pain and inflammation.

Besides, wheat, milk products, and meats, other foods high on the list of culprits for triggering arthritic symptoms include eggs, sugar and sugar substitutes, saturated fatty foods, and caffeinated drinks. It is best to eat whole, organic foods rather than processed ones.

These examples show how changing the diet can turn into a very important treatment in reversing or preventing arthritis, as well as many other disease processes. If diet can directly contribute to a disease, a change in that diet should take care of the problem. This should make more sense than giving someone a drug that will only tell the brain "it does not hurt anymore". Pain protects naturally. If it does not hurt, it does not mean that the problem disappears. It only means that we're continuing to destroy the joint–only we can't feel just how bad it really is.

Glucosamine and Chondroitin

The arthritic sufferer will find a variety of nutritional supplements on the market. However, what works for one, may not work for another. For actually stopping cartilage destruction and rebuilding the area, consider glucosamine sulphate. It is one of the eight essential sugars that the body requires in order to function properly.

Scientists have always known that sugar covers every cell in the body, but they thought it was all glucose and scraped it away to reach the protein they thought was the actual communicator for that cell. However, within the last fifteen years, they have found that actually the sugar coating directs traffic into the cell. Since they also thought that all sugars entering the body transformed into glucose, they found another surprise. Each tissue has its own predominant essential sugar.

As an essential sugar, glucosamine sulphate specifically targets cartilage and collagen fibres. Another sugar (but not an essential one) called chondroitin sulphate increases significantly the usefulness of glucosamine. We know both to as major building blocks of the water-loving proteoglycans, which branch off from the side of the cartilage and collagen fibres to increase their volume and ability to hold water. Since articular cartilage has no blood supply, all of its nourishment and lubrication come from the liquid that ebbs and flows as pressure to the joint is applied and released. Without this fluid, cartilage becomes malnourished and grows dry, thin, and more fragile.

Glucosamine is the key factor in determining how many proteoglycans the chondrocytes (cartilage cells) produce. Studies have shown that a high glucosamine content means more proteoglycans, with more water held in place. Low glucosamine content means fewer proteoglycans and less water in the area. Because glucosamine stimulates the production of key elements of the cartilage matrix and then protects it, it can actually help the body to repair damaged or eroded cartilage, which, in turn, helps to reduce pain and improve joint function.

Antioxidants destroy dangerous free radicals, which cause disease. Also anti-inflammatory, antioxidants include such vitamins as A (in the form of caratenoids), C, and E, as well as other nutrients.

- Vitamin C is a water-soluble vitamin lacking in those with arthritis, particularly those with Rheumatoid Arthritis. It is a nutrient vital for many body functions, including cartilage and bone formation. When combined with bioflavonoids, it helps to strengthen collagen, which cannot do its work at all without the presence of vitamin C. Using pharmaceuticals will rapidly deplete vitamin C in the body. Since the body eliminates this vitamin quickly, including the timed-release forms, you should take several smaller doses throughout the day instead of one large dose. Taking it along with vitamin E helps to reduce inflammation and speed joint healing.

* Vitamin D is essential for the formation, growth, and maintenance of bones and necessary for the absorption of calcium. Both work wonders in helping to reduce the effects of osteoarthritis.

* Vitamin E is depleted when inflammation is present. Studies have shown that, by taking 400-600 mg per day, a patient can reduce osteoarthritis symptoms. Taking a mixed form of vitamin E containing alpha, beta, delta, gamma tocophenols and tocotrienols is seven times better than taking the popular form of d-alpha tocophenol alone.

We can choose from many antioxidants, and can find them in a variety of natural foods. Those who eat high levels of antioxidants show a much slower rate of joint deterioration, particularly in the knees. Brightly coloured fruits and vegetables make the best sources of antioxidants.

B vitamins consist of a large family. Pantothenic acid (B5) aids in tissue repair. Those with Rheumatoid Arthritis often show a deficiency of this vitamin. Some nutrition-oriented doctors now prescribe as much as 1000 mg of B5 to help with morning stiffness, general disability, and pain. Another, B6, helps reduce swelling and joint stiffness. Several other nutrients, including glucosamine and chondroitin sulphates, require B6 for assimilation into the body

Niacin (B3) can help increase joint mobility, improve muscle strength, and reduce fatigue; but it requires high doses. Therefore, you should take those doses under the supervision of a knowledgeable medical professional since an excess of one B vitamin could cause a deficiency of others. Experts also recommend patients take a good multiple B vitamin along with any isolated others. B vitamins have proven to help arthritic patients, even in very small amounts.

Capsicum, one of the most widely used spices in the world, is found in cayenne or other hot peppers. Those in Central and South America use it to increase circulation and aid digestion, and now we know it for its temporary analgesic and anti-inflammatory effects. Shown to act through a specific receptor on pain fibres, capsicum decreases the production and action of substance-P, a chemical released from nerve fibres in response to pain. It mediates an inflammatory response by causing blood vessel dilation and the release of histamine from mast cells.

At first, capsicum actually increases the release of substance-P, which feels like a burning sensation, whether in the mouth or on the skin. Later, substance-P production greatly decreases, reducing the overall pain and inflammation response. Originally, we thought that capsicum affected only those fibres that conduct the pain message from the skin to the CNS. However, we now believeit has a wider effect on all sensory nerves, playing a central role in the spinal cord, where substance-P acts as a neurotransmitter for pain stimuli.

Most forms of capsicum are administered via a cream and applied topically over the arthritic, or painful areas. The skin contains many small nerve branches that lead back to the main "trunks" of the nerve. When we apply capsicum to a nerve branch, substance-P is depleted simultaneously in all connecting branches. This affects the joint. Patients must use it daily over a period of a couple of weeks before enough builds up in the system to cause a major reduction in pain.

Curcumin is the active ingredient in the spice turmeric and another herbal plant effective for arthritic symptoms. As a member of the ginger family, it has the same anti-inflammatory effects attributed to hydrocortisone and phenylbutazone. Curcumin has been used for centuries in India to treat inflammation and pain, as well as aiding in the digestive process, Some think it inhibits the breakdown and metabolism of cortisone by the liver, which would increase the amount of circulating cortisone in the body, thus, prolonging its effect. Curcumin appears to be less active in experimental animals without adrenal glands, indicating that the herb may also work by stimulating the release of adrenal corticosteroids.

DMSO (dimethyl sulfoxide) is a bi-product of the wood industry, and first introduced for therapeutic use in 1963. During the 1970s, doctors extensively prescribed DMSO in Russia to rheumatic patients. It's now widely used worldwide as a treatment for musculoskeletal inflammation.

DMSO is not found in the diet and patients must take it in supplemental form. The body easily absorbs and metabolises it. After ingestion, about 15 percent of DMSO is converted into MSM, one of its active components and one also used by arthritic sufferers. MSM increases the moisture-retaining and shock-absorbing qualities of joint cartilage and appears to decrease inflammation while providing building materials for collagen repair.

DMSO acts as an antioxidant by neutralizing oxidized

molecules in the body, particularly the joints. This ultimately has an effect on pain and inflammation in both inflammatory and non-inflammatory types of arthritis. It has proven effective when applied topically, lasting up to six hours. It offers the best results when the concentration ranges from 70 percent to 90 percent. In higher doses, the efficacy actually starts to decrease. The only side effect known is that it leaves a garlic taste in the mouth.

Essential Fatty Acids (EFA–omega oils) improve joint pain and stiffness by keeping the joints "lubricated" with "good" fats. Because of the modern diet, most people are 70 percent to 80 percent deficient. Symptoms of such deficiency include fatigue, dry skin and hair, acne, constipation, depression, bloating, and arthritis. EFAs are composed of **omega 3s**, which we can break down into three groups: alpha-linoleic acid (found in flax seeds, hempseeds, canola, soy, walnuts, and dark green leaves); stearidonic acids (found in black currants); and eicosapentaenoic acids (found in such cold-water fish as salmon, mackerel, sardines, and trout. Also a part of EFAs are **omega 6s,** which we can also break down into three groups: linolenic acids (LA) (found in the seeds of hempseeds, safflower, sunflower, soybeans, pumpkin, and sesame); gamma-linolenic acids (GLA), (found in the oils of borage seed or starflower, evening primrose, and black currant seeds); and arachidonic acids (found in meats and other animal products). GLA converts to a prostaglandin called E1, known to have anti-inflammatory effects. Another part of EFAs are **omegas 7 and 9** (oleic acids), widely abundant in olives, almonds, avocados, peanuts, cashews, and macadamia oils. Omega 7 is also found in coconut and palm oils. However, these fatty acids do not play a crucial role in the treatment of osteoarthritis, but omega 3 and 6 do.

Hempseeds offer an almost perfect balance between the omegas, more so than any other type of oil.

EFAs play a crucial role in determining which prostaglandins will be produced. They limit the availability of arachidonic acid (found in animal

products), which promotes the synthesis of "bad" prostaglandins involved in excessive inflammation production. By increasing EFA consumption, we can increase the production of the more beneficial prostaglandins. Clinical evidence for using EFAs in reducing the inflammation of arthritis is growing and proving to reduce pain and inflammation in the joint significantly.

EFAs also help to improve the good/bad ratio of cholesterol, soften skin and hair, and regulate bowel movements. The ideal ratio of omega 6 to omega 3 EFAs is about 3:1 or 4:1. Grocery store oils and salad dressings contain only omega 6 oils. They do not offer the ideal ratio, with the average consumption being 15:1. Cold-pressed oils make up excellent sources of EFAs and can be used as salad dressings, added to blender fruit drinks, or simply taken "as is". However, do not cook with them as heat destroys their value. Extra virgin olive oil is best used for cooking.

Ginger root, a staple of traditional Chinese medicine for thousands of years, helps decrease pain and inflammation. Well over 1,300 species of ginger root belong to the Zingiberaceae family, but the most commonly used ones are *Zingiber officinale* and *Alpinia galanga* (Greater Galanga), a Siamese type of ginger. Ginger contains several hundred active ingredients, but the most recognized ones are a group of active constituents called oleoresins. Ginger not only aids in the digestive process, but also inhibits the prostaglandin enzymes that cause inflammation. It also does not cause any of the gastric irritation seen in pharmaceutical anti-inflammatories.

Manganese is a mineral antioxidant, important for the synthesis of cartilage components. Although a deficiency will go unnoticed for a long period, such a deficiency can ultimately contribute to osteoarthritis.

MSM (methylsulfonylmethane) is a naturally occurring sulfur-containing compound used as a structural building material for cartilage. It contains about 34 percent sulphur, and comes from DMSO (dimethyl sulfoxide), another arthritis supplement. However, when DMSO enters the body, only about 15 percent converts into MSM. You can find MSM in such foods as fruit, alfalfa, corn, tomatoes. Breast milk is the richest source. Unfortunately, MSM is very volatileloses its therapeutic effects when the food is cooked, processed, or stored.

SAM-e (S-adenosylmethionine) comes from a combination of the essential amino acid methionine with ATP (adenosyl-triphosphate), the body's major form of energy storage. It's essentially three phosphate molecules attached together, forming a bond. If we break this bond, it leaves a di-phosphate and a single phosphate, releasing energy. The body uses this energy for every reaction that takes place, including muscle contractions, nerve impulse conductions, heartbeats, or antibody creations.

This combination of ATP and methionine increases the manufacture of certain cartilage components called proteoglycans. Blood levels of proteoglycans rise following supplementation with SAM-e. Just as with glucosamine and chondroitin sulfates, SAM-e also has a beneficial effect on cartilage. It also restores, indirectly reducing inflammation by reducing the destructive process.

Several studies have indicated that when patients consumed 1200 mg of SAM-e per day (400 mg 3 times a day); they experience a significant reduction in pain, stiffness, and other arthritic symptoms, rivalling that of several different NSAIDs. However, the price of the supplement deters patients, often causing people to bypass it entirely or to take a smaller dose. Not only does SAM-e help keep the joints healthy and strong by providing building materials to replace worn down cartilage, but it also helps indirectly to decrease the pain and inflammation of a joint through this repair. SAM-e does have one side effect. It appears to have anti-depressant properties and may elevate mood in those depressed because of chronic pain! All of this comes without hurting the body, while pharmaceutical anti-depressants cannot make the same claim.

Selenium is an antioxidant mineral found lacking in those with Rheumatoid Arthritis. These people seem to have an abnormality in their metabolism that affects the absorption of several nutrients, including this trace mineral. When they take Selenium with vitamin E, the effects of selenium are enhanced.

Zinc is a vital nutrient required by every cell in the body and necessary for the absorption and assimilation of many nutrients into the body. It's a vital co-factor involved in over 200 different enzyme reactions, as well as assisting in the production of several hormones.

We need zinc for cross-linking and regeneration of connective tissue in cartilage. Tests show that zinc metabolism is altered in those with arthritis, particularly Rheumatoid Arthritis. Zinc can successfully treat RA. Supplementation results in a slight decrease in pain and inflammation.

Zinc also helps heal wounds and works beneficially on the immune system, especially on colds and flu. The mineral, found abundantly in muscle tissue, plays an important role in health and maintenance. As an antioxidant, it helps to increase the function of the enzyme superoxide dismutase, which subsequently causes a reduction in free radical attacks on cellular structures and, therefore, decreases inflammation. Since zinc influences so many enzyme reactions and helps to assimilate other nutrients, its success in the area of muscle repair stands to reason as nutrients help the body repair itself. High doses of zinc can interfere with copper absorption and vice versa, and decrease immune function, however. You can find zinc in such foods as pumpkin seeds, almonds, ginger root, rye bread, oysters, and shellfish.

Zyflamend comes from herbs, and many arthritic sufferers find it useful in reducing the pain of inflammation. Scientists also found it has another benefit–reducing prostate cancer cells. Zyflamend consists of about a dozen different herbal extracts and offers more activity than that exerted by curcumin, the active ingredient in turmeric.

Much more information exists on the subject of arthritis and using diet to improve its condition. Many alternative therapies present themselves, but offer only temporary relief. However, dietary changes get to the root of the problem so that the body can heal itself permanently – not only of arthritis, but also of so many other conditions that plague the human race.

You can get all of these products online or via your local health food or vitamin suppliers.

Chapter 4

Recipes

Food plays an important role in everybody's life. Without food, we cannot survive. However, food also causes, or triggers, many diseases and allergies. Rheumatoid Arthritis is one of them. Remember the saying "We are what we eat?" Over the years I've adopted a firm belief in this philosophy. By a process of elimination I notice that some foods can directly affect the pain levels I experience. I aim to pass on that knowledge to you.

The arthritic cannot stand for long periods to prepare fresh food, so he soon becomes a convenience food junkie, often favouring microwave meals or tinned processed foods. Many books on the market today offer fancy recipes that take hours to prepare, making them an impossible dream to the pain-riddled arthritic, forcing him back to inadequate meals. Being a sufferer myself, I know what it's like to look at these fancy recipes and sigh when you read the one-hour preparation time. I considered those facts for this book. I know you cannot stand for hours preparing food, but I also know that you can make healthy, tasty dishes in a less time—and like it.

Did you know?

The most commonly observed vitamin and mineral deficiencies in patients with RA are folic acid, vitamin C, vitamin D, vitamin B_6, vitamin B_{12}, vitamin E, folic acid, calcium, magnesium, zinc and selenium.

In this chapter, we aim to provide a solution to that dilemma with recipes that take no more than thirty minutes to prepare and offer nutrition and affordability.

The basic food requirements remain the same for all people, whether sick or well: eating five pieces of fruit (arthritics should avoid citrus fruits due to the acid) and vegetables, cutting down on saturated fats (easily recognisable as they remain hard at room temperature, i.e. butter, lard, suet and fat on meat), drinking plenty of water, and most important, eating a fresh green salad daily. Following these requirements provides our bodies with vital nutrients and minerals that give us a feeling of well-being. That good feeling does not come through processed foods.

It's important to adopt a low fat diet as many arthritic patients also suffer from associated diseases, such as angina, high blood pressure and kidney problems, due in part to the illness and the side effects of years of drug-taking. We don't know a cure for arthritis, but by trying the recipes in this book and following the advice given by the experts, you can lose the pain and control the illness yourself, without the need of harmful drugs. Remember, eating wholesome, healthy food does not mean starving yourself or craving foods.

Foods that can affect your arthritis and we classify as

nightshade vegetables. This list unfortunately includes potatoes, tomatoes, eggplant, red and green peppers and paprika. We know that they affect 1 or 2 percent of Rheumatoid Arthritis suffers. An American horticulturist, Norman F. Childers, developed the theory in the 1940s that nightshades could exacerbate RA symptoms. He found that eliminating foods of the nightshade family cured his arthritis. He believed that eating nightshade foods results in "a build-up of cholinesterase inhibiting glycoalkaloids and steroids and may cause inflammation, muscle spasms, pain, and stiffness." If you notice your pain increases after consuming these nightshade vegetables, then exclude them from your diet. I have included them in some of these recipes for those not affected by them, but those of you who are affected, please do not despair. You can easily replace them with pasta, rice or extra salad. These recipes serve two to four people, unless otherwise noted.

Pan Fried Chicken & Spicy Couscous

Ingredients

- 1 pound skinless, boneless, chicken breasts, chopped into strips
- 1-1/3 cups couscous grains
- 1/4 cup lemon juice (fresh or bottled)
- 2 tablespoons extra virgin olive oil
- 1 red chilli, finely chopped (optional)
- 2 medium carrots, shredded
- 2-1/2 teaspoons ground cumin seeds
- 1-1/2 teaspoon ground ginger
- 3/4 teaspoon salt
- 1/2 teaspoon black pepper
- 1/4 cup currants or raisins
- 1/4 cup chopped coriander

(For those who require a vegetarian alternative, omit the chicken, use all the spices in the couscous mixture, but then add 2 cups of cooked chickpeas to the couscous in the final step. It still tastes great!)

Method

Preheat the frying pan (the oil should sizzle when it hits the pan). In a small bowl, combine 1 teaspoon cumin and ginger, ¼ teaspoon salt, and half the black pepper. Rub mixture into the chicken so that covers chicken evenly. Fry for 4 minutes per side, or until just cooked through.

While the chicken fries, combine in a large saucepan the water, remaining cumin, ginger, and black pepper and bring to a boil over high heat. Add the couscous. Remove pan from heat, cover, and let stand 5 minutes, until couscous has softened. Fluff with a fork. Adding a knob of butter at this stage adds a velvety sheen to the couscous and tastes great, too.

In a large bowl, whisk together remaining 1/2 teaspoon salt, lemon juice, and oil. Add chicken, couscous, chilli, carrots, currants, and coriander, and toss to combine. Serve at room temperature or chilled.

This makes a great addition to a picnic or served with a BBQ as a side dish in the summer. Serve with iced lemon tea for a wonderful meal.

Welsh Rarebit

The name "Welsh Rabbit" confuses even the British, because it's always consisted of only delicious melted cheese on toasted bread. You can modify it by adding vegetables of your choice. Here I offer the basic recipe which you can modify any way you want to.

Ingredients

2 tablespoons butter
3 cups aged cheddar, shredded
½ cup ale or beer
2 egg yolks, beaten
1 teaspoon English dry mustard, ground
1 teaspoon cayenne pepper
1 teaspoon Worcestershire sauce.
Salad leaves for serving

Method

Start with all ingredients, except cheese, at room temperature. Using a double boiler, add all the ingredients except for the cheese, bringing it to a gentle simmer. Add cheese a little at a time, and stir until the cheese melts and sauce thickens. Spread evenly over the bread and grill until lightly browned. Serve with crisp salad and enjoy.

Onion Omelette with Salad

Ingredients

1 tablespoon olive oil
2 large red onions, chopped
1 red pepper, diced
2 large eggs
Whites of 5 large eggs
1/2 teaspoon salt
1/4 teaspoon black pepper
Fresh salad leaf selection
Lemon juice (optional)

Method

Heat the oil over a medium flame in a large non-stick frying pan. Gradually add the onions and red pepper and cook, stirring frequently, until the onions soften and brown, about 5 minutes.

Whisk together the eggs, egg whites, salt, and black pepper until well blended in a bowl.

Remove the pan from the heat and pour the egg mixture on top of the vegetable mixture. Cover, and cook until the eggs are just set in the centre, about 10 minutes over a low heat.

Place salad leaves in a bowl, drizzle with olive oil and a little lemon juice (optional) season lightly and serve with slices of the omelette, either hot or cold.

Tuna Pasta with Fresh Baby Spinach

Ingredients

12 ounces whole wheat pasta (any shape you want)
1 tablespoon extra-virgin olive oil
1 small onion, chopped
1-1/4 pounds tomatoes, coarsely chopped
1 pound baby spinach, coarsely chopped
1 can albacore tuna in brine or water, drained
3 tablespoons grated Parmesan cheese
1 teaspoon salt
1/4 teaspoon pepper

Method

Cook the pasta of your choice according to package directions. Drain.

In large non-stick frying pan, heat oil over medium heat. Add onion and cook gently, until softened, about 5 minutes.

Add the chopped tomatoes, and cook until they begin to soften, about 5 minutes.

Increase heat to high; add spinach and cook until spinach just wilts, about 2 to 3 minutes. Add drained pasta, tuna, Parmesan, salt & pepper to taste, and toss gently to combine. Serve hot.

Scallops with Brown Rice

Ingredients

3 tablespoons light soy sauce
3 tablespoons white wine vinegar
1 tablespoon dark sesame oil
1-1/2 teaspoons Dijon mustard
8 ounces wholemeal (brown) rice
2 carrots, shredded
1 chilli pepper, cut into 2-inch matchsticks
2 teaspoons olive oil
1 pound queen scallops, halved horizontally
4 spring onions, thinly sliced
2 tablespoons minced fresh root ginger
2 cloves garlic, crushed
2 teaspoons toasted sesame seeds

Method

In large bowl, mix the soy sauce, vinegar, sesame oil, mustard, and 3 tablespoons of water.

Cook the rice according to package directions and drain. Add to bowl along with carrots and chilli and toss to combine.

In large non-stick frying pan, gently fry the scallops for 1 minute. Add remaining ingredients cook 1 minute or until scallops are just cooked through. Add scallop mixture to bowl with rice, tossing to combine.

To serve, divide salad among 2-4 plates, sprinkle with sesame seeds, Serve warm with crusty bread and butter.

Waldorf Salad with Roast Chicken

Ingredients

1 pound skinless, boneless cooked chicken breast
3/4 cup plain fat-free yogurt
1/4 cup low fat sour cream
1 tablespoon cider vinegar
2 teaspoons Dijon mustard
1/2 teaspoon salt
2 red apples, cut into 1/2-inch cubes
2 celery sticks, halved lengthwise and thinly sliced
1/4 cup walnuts, coarsely chopped
6 cups fresh crisp lettuce hearts
1/4 cup chicken stock

Method:

Cut chicken breasts into bite-size pieces.

In large bowl, whisk together 1/4 cup chicken stock, yogurt, sour cream, vinegar, mustard, and salt. Add chicken, apples, celery, and walnuts, tossing well to combine.

Add lettuce, toss, and serve with warm crusty bread.

Triple Berry Salad Dessert

Ingredients

1/4 cup fresh orange juice
2 tablespoons balsamic vinegar
2 tablespoons rich dark brown sugar
1/8 teaspoon pepper
1/8 teaspoon allspice
3 cups chopped strawberries
1 cup raspberries
1 cup blackberries
1/2 cup toasted walnut pieces

Method

Whisk together orange juice, vinegar, sugar, pepper, and allspice in a bowl. Add strawberries, raspberries, and blackberries and toss to coat.

To serve, spoon berry mixture into small bowls and sprinkle walnuts on top. Add a splash of cream for that extra special treat!

Banana Muesli Breakfast for Two

Ingredients

2 tablespoons rolled oats
2 bananas, chopped or sliced
1 tablespoon of honey
1/2 cup natural low fat yoghurt
Chopped nuts – optional

Method

Mix oats banana and honey together in a bowl. Add yogurt and stir thoroughly, making sure you do not break banana. Spoon into bowls and eat immediately.

Fruit Salad for Two

Ingredients

A few grapes, halved
1 sliced banana
1 apple chopped
Lemon juice

Method

Combine all the ingredients in a bowl and stir. Squeeze juice of half a lemon over the fruit to prevent discolouring. Serve with cream and slice of wholemeal toast.

Grilled Haddock

Ingredients

1 medium sized haddock fillet, skinless and boneless
1 tablespoon melted margarine or butter
1/2 cup of wholemeal flour
Salt and pepper to season flour

Method

Wash and trim the fish. Brush both sides of fish with the melted butter. Toss fish in the seasoned flour until completely coated. Place under a preheated grill and cook gently for 15 minutes turning as required.

Serve with fresh salad, wholemeal bread and butter and lemon wedge.

From the Author

Feel free to contact me at contact@suzanne-harris.com for recipe updates, all of which will come out soon in my Arthritics' Cookbook!

I hope the information in this book can help you on your quest to find better health. It will not cure your arthritis, which is not curable, but it does show you an alternative route to prescribed medication. These methods may not suit everyone and perhaps it works best for you alongside your traditional medicine. It's your illness and your body; make your own choices and do what works for you.

To order additional copies of
Rheumatoid Arthritis: The Alternate Route

Name ____

Address ______________________________________

____

____

$9.95 x ____________ copies = ___________

Sales Tax ___________________
(Texas residents add 8.25% sales tax)

Please add $3.50 postage and handling _ _______

Total amount due: _____________________________

Please send check or money order for books to:

WordWright.biz, Inc.
WordWright Business Park
46561 State Highway 118
Alpine, TX 79830

For a complete catalog of books or
to order online,
visit our site at
http://www.WordWright.biz

Printed in the United States
49707LVS00001B/25-27

9 781932 196870